INTRODUCTION TO BECOMING AND REMAINING RUGBYFIT

James Haskell
Wasps and England

INTRODUCTION TO BECOMING AND REMAINING RUGBYFIT

ISBN 978-1-5262-0213-0

First published 2016 © James Haskell Health & Fitness

Acknowledgements

Susie Haskell
Jonathan Haskell
Edward Haskell
Bob Waite — BW Design
Matt Pell — Matt&Dan Studio
Dan Bartha — Matt&Dan Studio
Baris Kasikirik — Olusur Basim Hizmetleri
Louise Robinson — Backtofrontdesign
Omar Meziane — Executive Chef Great Britain Rowing

Plus anyone who we have inadvertently forgotten to credit or acknowledge

---

Design Team BW Design – Graphics & Text, Matt&Dan Studio – Branding & Art Direction, Backtofrontdesign – Pre-publication & Artwork. **Photography** Adrian Myers Photography, Tickle Media, Dave Rogers/Getty Images, Associated Press Images, IStock, Shutterstock, Christian Couzens Photography, Andy Hooper - Daily Mail, Richard Lane Photography, David Clerihew - RFU, Josh Cawthorn Photography.

JAMES HASKELL HEALTH & FITNESS HELPS YOU ACHIEVE A HEALTHIER AND FITTER LIFESTYLE We do this by delivering professional fitness and nutrition advice in a simple, clear and easy to understand format. In conjunction with the development of our own range of clean and certified sports supplements, this allows the individual to achieve the lifestyle balance, which is right for them. All of our Supplements and Training books are exclusively created and produced in Britain. JHHF is proud to support and work with British talent, in order to fully utilise the great skill-set this Country boasts

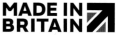

INDEX

Cover picture Adrian Myers

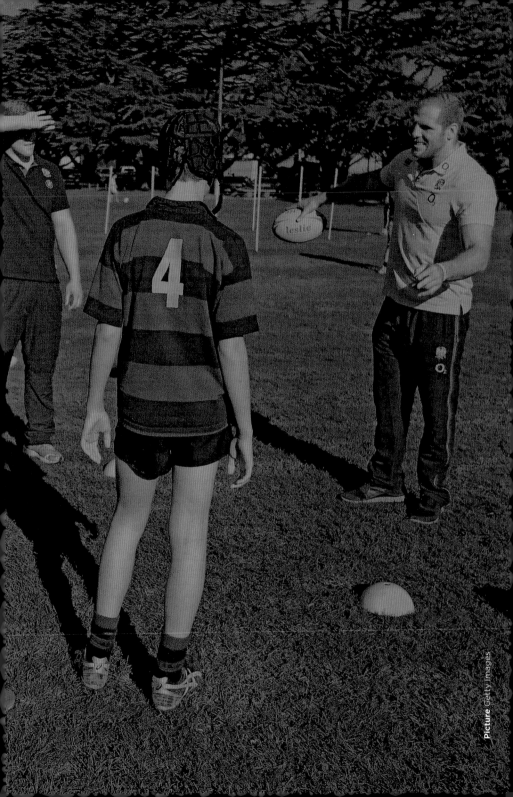

REAP THE FRUITS OF JAMES'S MULTI CULTURAL EXPERIENCES

James Haskell exhortation has always been to train for rugby with your brain, as well as your body. He has bravely and boldly chosen to experience a multi-cultural rugby life, playing in all four of the top professional leagues in World Rugby; France, England, Japan and Super 15 rugby in New Zealand. Not to mention the small matter of 66 tests for England. He has trained under some of the Sport's greatest coaches and consequently has soaked up all the unique and different experiences, in the quest for the perfect conditioning package, of lifestyle, sports science and all the technical aspects.

"I have to say James Haskell's RugbyFit Book is a classic."

It is true to say that all these career experiences are now crammed into his new project, the James Haskell RugbyFit book. He is always inundated with questions from players of all standards and aspirations, questions on all aspects of preparation to play the greatest game. His vast accumulated store of knowledge now reside in one publication and anyone who aspires to improvement and to improving their game out of sight, together with those of us who coach hopeful youngsters, will be delving into that store.

"James Haskell RugbyFit Book is concise, precise, cutting-edge, and sympathetic."

There are several features which I find very comforting. Haskell demolishes the idea that sheer size and endless heavy weight-training should be everything in rugby. He holds up as the perfect training balance the New Zealand idea that around 65% of training time should be devoted to rugby and skills and 35% to the gym and allied work. Also, you do not have to be a world-class powerlifter to complete all the exercises in the book. Granted, some of the drills and exercises can sound a little scary. The Romanian dead-lift. The Lizard crawl. The Bulgarian split-squat. But the clarity of Haskell's explanations, his summaries of the key points in performing all the parts of the plan, will soon re-assure you. He does not lay out a plan to avoid the hard work, far from it.

"This is heads-up preparation for rugby, and it will do you a world of good."

But this book is not for obsessives, or for the muscle-bound. It is for rugby players, and on every page, we learn where each stage relates to the actual game. He also outlines rest and recovery protocols, recommends sharp sessions of no more than an hour. He suggests what time in the week and the season calls for what kinds of sessions.

James Haskell RugbyFit Book is concise, precise, cutting-edge, and sympathetic. We all treasure heads-up rugby. This is heads-up preparation for rugby, and it will do you a world of good.

Stephen Jones - Rugby Writer of the Year
The Sunday Times

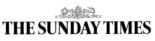

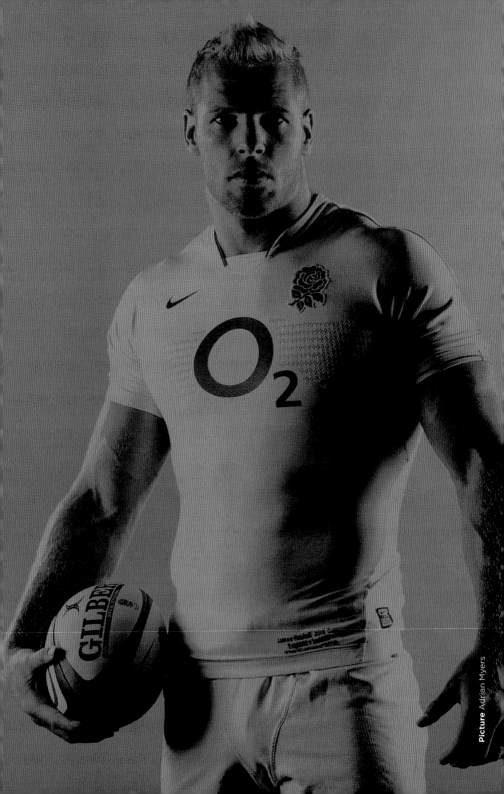

THE INTRODUCTION TO RUGBYFIT

Whether you are a loyal follower or new to James Haskell Health & Fitness (JHHF) we promise you won't be disappointed in the contents of our first comprehensive rugby book.

It has been designed to provide you with the broadest possible introduction to all the key areas with which you will need to become acquainted and engaged. It will set you firmly on the path to becoming #RugbyFit.

If, having tried the initial package, you want to progress into more specialist training areas then very soon there will be focussed packages available, to help improve those specific areas and accelerate your development both as an athlete and a rugby player.

The past 12 years of James's rugby career have gone into the making of this book. He has been lucky enough to have played around the world, working with some of the best coaches and experts in their respective fields of fitness, nutrition and medical science. Now it is time to share this unique information and insider knowledge with you.

James Haskell Health & Fitness helps you achieve a healthier and fitter lifestyle. We do this delivering professional fitness and nutrition advice in a simple, clear and easy to understand format. In conjunction with the development of our own range of clean and certified sports supplements, this allows the individual to achieve the lifestyle balance, which is right for them.

We want you to achieve your fitness goals whatever they might be. So make sure you stay in touch with us and let us know how things are going. We always love to receive your tweets and photos and will of course re-post wherever we can.

Twitter @jameshaskellhf
Instagram @jameshaskellhf
Face book jameshaskellhealthandfitness

If you have any questions then the team at JHHF are always there to try to help and answer them as quickly as they can. Please email all questions to askhask@jameshaskell.com

Our mantra is TRAIN LIKE A PRO and our goal is to get you doing just that in as short a time as possible.

Thank you again for your purchase and good luck getting #RugbyFit

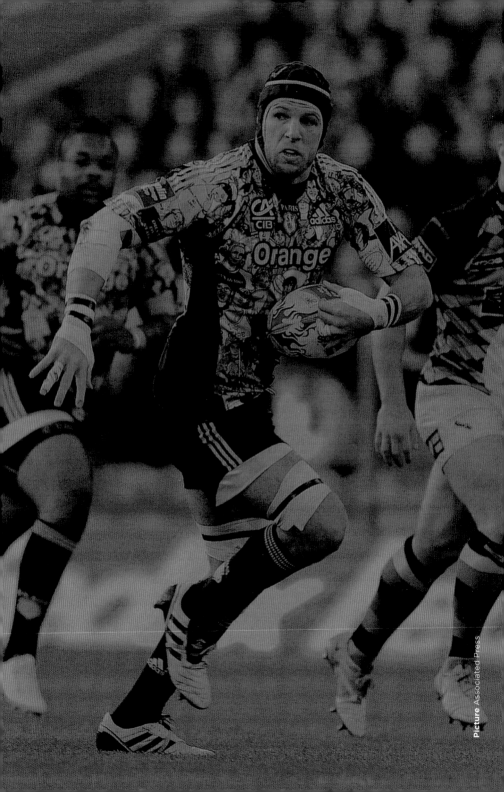

PLEASE READ THE IMPORTANT NOTES BELOW BEFORE CONTINUING

INTRODUCTION

This package has been designed to start you on your journey to becoming RugbyFit by introducing and teaching you the basic, foolproof methods you need to adopt to be successful at rugby training. By developing the extensive skillset needed to become a successful rugby player, you will in turn develop yourself into a successful athlete.

These are sessions and approaches, which have been tried and tested by James throughout his career and are the current methods he still uses today to stay RugbyFit.

If you are a young player looking to get started then this package is certainly for you.

However the package is also ideal for anyone looking to step-up their training and take it to a new level; be it a club player, university player or even an amateur looking to take things more seriously.

As detailed in the welcome section on page 7, this is a broad cover-all approach. However once you know exactly where you want your subsequent focus to be, additional, bespoke programmes covering a series of particular training areas and focus, will shortly be available from www.jameshaskell.com.

However as a start we are going to look at the following areas:

- Warm-up
- HIIT Cardio
- Resistance Training
- Bodyweight Training
- Power Endurance
- Running Fitness

- Rugby Specific Conditioning
- Core Rugby Skill Drills
- Recovery
- Nutrition
- Supplements

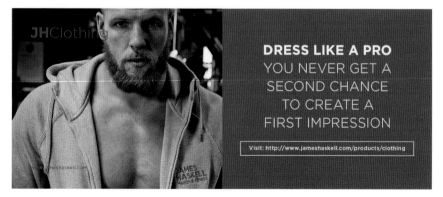

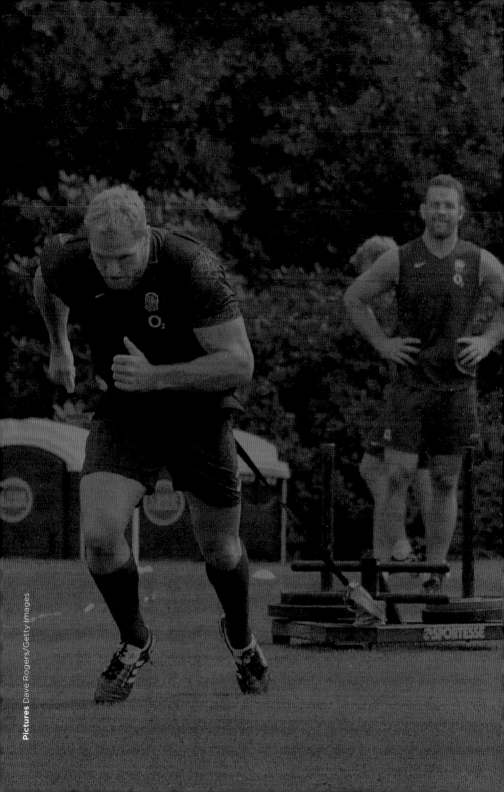

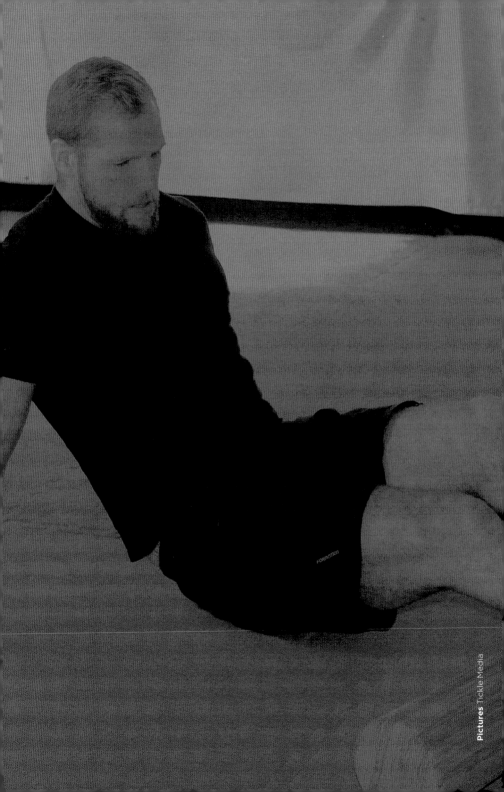

THE TRAINING PRINCIPLES BEHIND THIS BOOK

James firmly believes, as does Warren Gatland the Wales Coach, who famously introduced high intensity training to Wasps all those years ago; that a training session doesn't have to be overly long. Instead it needs to be intense and focussed. This is the core principle behind our approach.

A really important thing to note, is before every session we suggest in this programme (bar the recovery information) you will need to perform a proper warm-up to raise your core body temperature (CBT). We will refer to this warm-up as 'the CBT warm-up'. See the warm-up section below for more information.

TRAINING TYPE/STYLE:
1. WARM-UP

Injuries are common when training. However they are mainly due to human error and therefore can be minimised with the right care and approach. Always undertake a proper warm-up, each and every time you start to exercise and/or train. It is the single most important corner stone foundation and safeguard you can create for yourself.

Common causes of injury often include:

* Insufficient or worse still, no proper warm-up procedure
* Lifting using incorrect technique or bad form
* Lifting weights which are too heavy
* Failing to stretch enough throughout the week

James says:
"Having played rugby for a long time and being very inflexible by nature, I often need to do a pre warm-up to my warm-up. One of the ways I do this is either some band work to open up the muscles, or I use a foam roller. I don't go mad with this; I focus on my back and major muscle groups. This isn't for everyone, but it can be very useful"

I have made a video about foam rolling – visit
www.youtube.com/theJamesHaskell

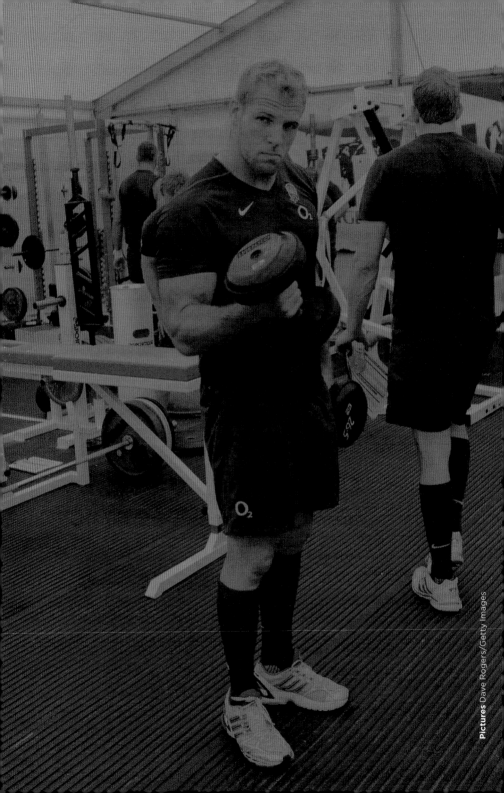

2. HIIT CARDIO

HIIT stands for "High Intensity Interval Training", with the aim to accelerate fat burning whilst retaining lean muscle mass.

High Intensity Interval Training involves a series of very high intensity exercises, working to 90%+ of your maximum heart rate. For example, exercises based on sprinting, battle ropes, bodyweight work and the like, followed by a series of low intensity exercises, such as walking, steady peddling or rest.

So the pattern we want is High Intensity - Low Intensity.

HIIT for most people will more likely help preserve lean muscle tissue as opposed to long spurts of cardio. Plus mentally, a 20 minute HIIT session is far easier to knuckle down and do, than spending hours pounding the treadmill.

3. RESISTANCE TRAINING

The key to getting bigger or being stronger is basically all about your time spent in the gym.

Lifting weights or using bodyweight will both help with your physical development.

The Resistance Training [RT] sessions outlined within this package are based around "time under tension" work, which is all about building muscle.

4. BODYWEIGHT WORK

Bodyweight work is a really useful tool to whatever you are hoping to do when it comes to training. Its not just for beginners its for everyone. If you want to get into training then this is a great place to start, it reduces the risk of injury and allows you to build a good foundation.

Once you have this cracked you can then progress on to weights. Bodyweight work can also be done anywhere, so it is great for home users, holidays and staying fit on the go. There is no need for a gym.

5. POWER ENDURANCE

This is a combination of circuit exercises used to mimic the range of physical sensations and fatigue you will experience during a game.

Rugby is not about long distance endurance; it's about being able to perform a multitude of jobs continuously for short bursts of time. These jobs range from swiftly getting on and off the floor, to clearing out rucks, sprinting, tackling, jogging, lifting, rucking and so forth.

For these power endurance sessions, we have put together elements which mimic these situations. For example we use weights, tyre flips, shuttles, tug of war and so forth, to induce you into the same state of fatigue you would experience in a game.

6. RUNNING FITNESS

These sessions are designed to increase your overall running fitness. The sessions are based on the kind of running intensity you will experience playing rugby. They are also there to build a base fitness level.

Rugby players, whilst covering a huge amount of ground, are not marathon runners. So there is no point in training to run for miles. The sessions will mimic the intensity you find in a game. They will also help you build stamina and an endurance fitness base.

7. RUGBY SPECIFIC CONDITIONING

These are sessions which are purposely developed for rugby players and will condition your body to deal with the kind of fitness you will require on the field of play.

The idea behind this kind of work is to replicate the intensity and physicality of tackles, running and getting quickly back off the floor and into a defensive or attacking position. This is also key for testing your rugby skills under pressure.

These will mainly be pitch based and will require the use of some specialist equipment.

8. CORE SKILL DRILLS

The core skills of rugby are drills like passing, breakdown work, tackling, managing highballs and choosing the correct running lines. This is the most important area of the whole package and will help you develop the skills required to become a competent rugby player.

While the idea is to give you a taste of all the different types of training you can do, it's important to remember to consistently practice the skills of the sport you are undertaking, in this case rugby.

9. RECOVERY

Recovery is essential to training and progressing in your chosen sport or activity. We take you through some of the best recovery protocols that are available for you to use. There is not one miracle technique that works in isolation; you need to use things in combination, which combine different elements in order to get the best results.

Diet and nutrition is also a really important area that very often gets neglected when it comes to recovery. It can affect you physically, mentally and performance wise if you don't get it right. Fuel your body correctly with healthy sources of protein, carbohydrates and fat to yield ultimate performance and maximise your recovery.

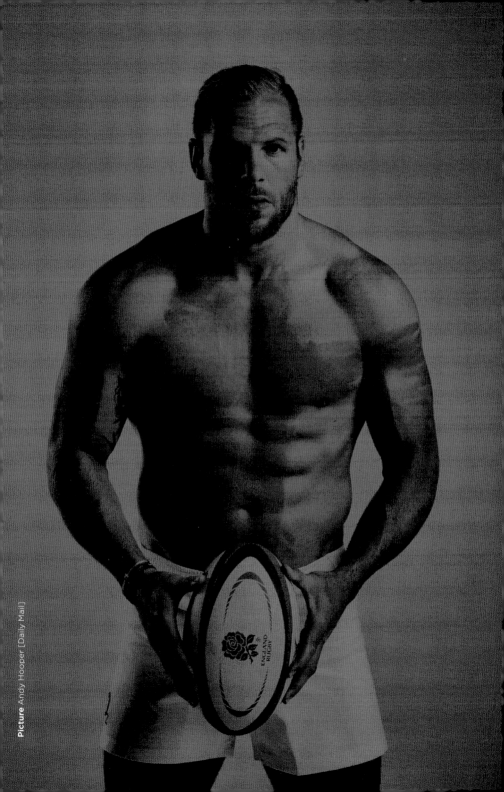

POINTS AND QUESTIONS TO ADDRESS BEFORE WE BEGIN

1. PHYSICAL SIZE

Currently there is a huge obsession amongst aspiring young players and the rugby public at large, in believing that you have to be a massive individual to play rugby. This is most definitely not the case. So the obsession needs to end here!

The most important elements you need to be a good rugby player are great core skills, speed, power and strength. Size is a by-product of some of these, but no one got anywhere by just being massive.

Some of the most difficult players to tackle in world rugby are certainly not the biggest, but what they do have is quick feet, power, strength and great core skills. That is why they are so devastating when carrying. Just being huge won't take you to the next level.

This also works the other way round when it comes to the best defenders in the world. If you are constantly missing tackles, don't assume it's down to your size. That is an easy excuse, the reason could well be down to your tackle technique and how you execute it.

With this in mind, everything you should do on your journey to becoming a rugby player, or improving as a rugby player, should be centred around developing and perfecting the core skills of the game.

By these I mean:

- Passing
- Footwork
- Tackle Technique
- Aerial Work
- Ball Carrying
- Breakdown Work
- Set Piece
- Game Awareness

If you aren't touching upon one of these areas every day then you are going wrong.

On a pro-rata basis, it is far more important you spend time on these critical core skills than in the gym.

If I could only give one piece of advice to anyone out there, it would be to allocate an extra 10 minutes every day to work on one of these areas. Then rotate the following day.

James says:
"Practicing my core skills is what I have done for the last twelve years and indeed still do after every training session."

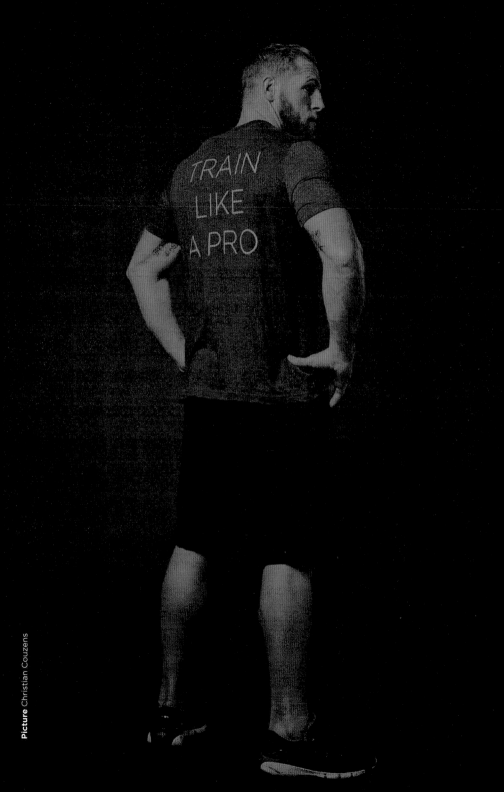

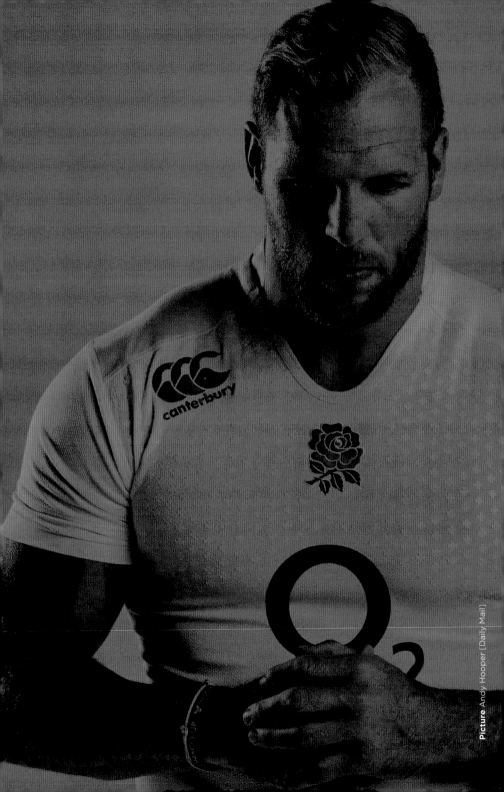

2. HOW DO I STAND OUT IN A TRIAL? (A question we are tweeted all the time)

The answer is definitely not about how much you can bench or how big you are. Instead, it is - can you clearly demonstrate excellent technical ability and utilise the correct core skills as effectively as possible?

As a player, you need to understand exactly what it is you do best. You might be an awesome ball carrier or a smashing tackler - you have to make sure you bring those points of difference out on the field during play.

At the same time as constantly striving to improve on what you already do well, you also need to focus on your weak points. However hard you try, there will always be areas of your game that are stronger than others; the key is to balance improving your weaknesses with refining your areas of excellence.

If you keep getting brushed-off in the tackle it is probably not because you are too small, but because your technique is either off or fundamentally poor.

If you don't make the gain line then you need to look at how you carry the ball into contact. It could be down to body position, lack of footwork, or over use of it and what sort of running lines you adopt.

You need to focus on these aspects before you get carried away with weights. If you understand these fundamental points then you can look to improve yourself physically as the next step.

James says:
"Trying to build strength and size at the expense of good rugby technique is not the answer and should definitely not dictate your approach to training."

3. WHY IS FITNESS SO IMPORTANT FOR RUGBY PLAYERS?

The simple answer is if you're fit and in shape you're more likely to make the right decisions at the right time.

If you're tired you can't think properly, thus you are more likely to make a mistake. People most often make mistakes under fatigue, which is the point behind some of the training we do in modern rugby. With the advancement in technology, we wear for both club and country GPS vests with heart rate monitors to track everything we do, to monitor our physical ability and workrate.

Vast data has been collected on the intensity of actual matches, so training needs to replicate that level at times. If it doesn't, then you aren't effectively prepared for what you have to do when it comes to the pressure of a real game.

Training will be structured to reach these levels a couple of times of week; to ensure boys test their skill sets under pressure. This is the thinking behind having a strong fitness base to ensure you test your skill sets under pressure. It should always be taken into account when preparing for a new season, trial, or any sort of competition.

James says:
"Fitness never gets easier, but if you are RugbyFit you will always find it much easier to make the right decisions and reduce the chances of making a mistake."

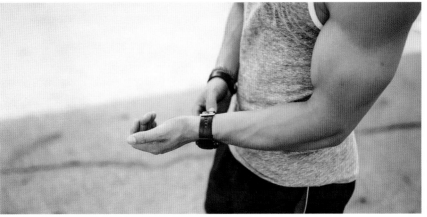

Picture Istock

4. ONE HOUR OF TRAINING IS ENOUGH!

When you are in the gym or doing any form of training, expect it to be hard work from the 'get-go', but also expect to be walking out no longer than an hour from starting. Even when the sessions are lifting-based, they are designed to be effective and get you training smarter and quicker.

Obviously not all sessions have to be super physically demanding, some will be mentally demanding in some form.

Pushing yourself both mentally and physically is what will make the difference and get you your results.

Taking two and half hours to do a rugby session is most definitely not the right way of doing things. If you or your club team spend anywhere close to this then immediately look to try and change things.

Your session plan should be clear and pre-planned, with the areas that need work being clearly defined. Then if you need to stay later and work on specialist areas plus your core skills, you know exactly what to do.

I would say as a maximum the sessions should never be longer than one hour and thirty minutes - including the warm-up. After this time period, you begin to experience heavy fatigue, which can impair your recovery, increase your risk of injury and halt your progress. There are no benefits that you will gain by training longer – you have to train smarter.

Most sessions in this programme will consist of a CBT (core body temperature) functional warm-up, based on getting you moving the natural way.

James says:
"These warm-ups are not a simple five minutes on an X-trainer. They are hard work and you should be puffing, hot and sweaty by the time you enter the gym floor. If you are doing a pitch session then the same applies. You need to get yourself properly warmed-up and moving."

5. PRE TRAINING ROUTINES

There are various different ways that people prepare for training sessions. A lot of it depends on whether you are training in the morning, afternoon, or a couple of times throughout the day.

I always start my day with a focus on hydration. I take this to the next level by using a pro-hydrate tablet in water. The idea is to provide your body with extra electrolytes and salts that you will have lost when sleeping. I am always very dehydrated in the mornings. If I don't address this I feel terrible and as a consequence under perform.

These are tailored to the level of salt that you lose when sweating. You can speak to the guys at the company www.myh2pro.com and get tested or have a look on our website www.jameshaskell.com to purchase the products to help you start to get this area right.

I also recommend taking one of my all natural, award winning, Informed Sport approved, pre training supplement tablets, Hades for men, Hella for women, thirty minutes before the start of your session to enhance focus and maximise performance. Available here www.jameshaskell.com

James says:
"Hades and Hella are great for boosting your training and performance. The feedback we have is amazing; people who use our supplements find they have none of the issues associated with other pre-trainers; such as head rushes, palpitations or the jitters. All you get with Hades and Hella is a sustained burst of energy, which helps you push yourself harder for longer, to get the results you want."

Have a look at both our website and social media for all the amazing feedback our products get. Twitter @jameshaskellhf. Instagram: jameshaskellhf.

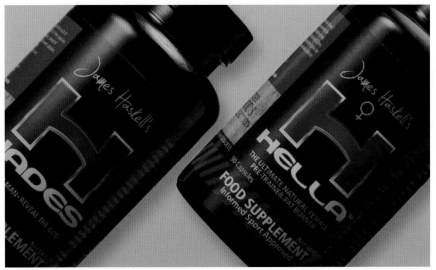

Picture Istock

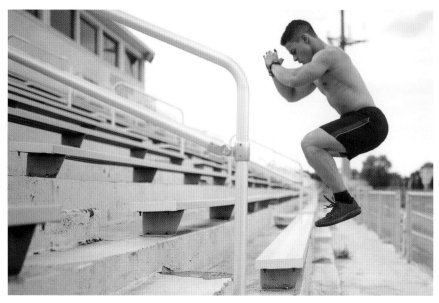

6. DURING YOUR WORKOUT

Make sure you stay hydrated throughout your training by drinking plenty of water. During training is when you can drink energy drinks such as Lucozade and Powerade. However, I would avoid drinking these types of drinks at any other time.

Like all the tips and tricks we suggest for you, it's really important you test these out when you have nothing at stake. For example don't try these things for the first time on game day, instead introduce them before a training session or before some light intensity work.

It is also important you test them a number of times to get a good idea of how they all work. But much more importantly, how they work for you. Everybody is different and thus reacts differently.

James says:
"Another option for you is to look to take Branch Chain Amino Acids, or known in their shortened form as BCAA'S. They help fuel your muscles during training so you don't go into a catabolic (muscle eating state) we will cover more about these in the Supplement section (page 83). I have said many times before it is not essential you take supplements or BCAA's but for the right person who wants to top things up, or has the requirement because of training load, they can play a very important role."

It is not essential you take these but they are known to have training benefits which a lot of people have acknowledged. A lot will depend on the quality of your diet.

See more about this in Nutrition (page 76).

LETS GET STARTED!

STEP 1 WHAT YOUR TRAINING WEEK SHOULD LOOK LIKE

In each section of this programme there is a suggestion as to the volume of training you should be doing during the season, pre-season and down time. I want to give you an example of a normal training week, which I would undertake based around a Saturday game. You will be able to see where to incorporate what training and when.

The following chart is based on the assumption you have played eighty minutes, or close to that, the weekend before, most likely on the Saturday. So Monday being your first day back, you would not be doing too many conditioning extras, unless of course you felt you needed them.

The suggestions I have made are only recommendations. Some of the sessions are optional and you can choose what works for you.

Pay close attention to your levels of fatigue, to avoid overworking and risking injury or set back. It is also important to listen to the advice of Coaches and Conditioners, who will be able to help you determine the most effective training plan for you.

Monday	Tuesday	Wednesday	Thursday	Friday	Saturday	Sunday
Recovery	Lower body weights	Recovery protocols	Power weights			Recovery protocols
Massage						
Short HiiT session if needed	Rugby session	Day off	Rugby session	Rugby session	Game day	Day off
Upper body weights / Body weight work	Core skill drills / contact based		Core skills practice	Core skills practice		
Short fitness top up if required	Short fitness top up if required	Physio / mat				
Recovery	Recovery		Recovery	Recovery		Physio / mat

If you only have limited game time at the weekend, or no game at all, then your training programme for the next week will naturally look a little different. The Monday would certainly contain some conditioning; either running, power endurance, HIIT, or a mixture of the three.

On Tuesday, you could do some extra work in the weights room, core skills and add in some extra conditioning if you feel the need.

Your non playing weekend would look like this:

Friday	Saturday	Sunday
Rugby	Power endurance	Recovery protocol
Weights top up (upper or lower)	Running fitness	Day off

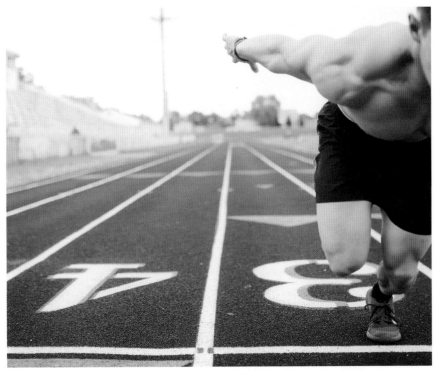

STEP 2 WARM UP

It is essential to remember a proper warm-up is absolutely key for injury avoidance and should never be skipped. This style of warm-up and the exercises shown have been approved by JHHF. But do remember, there are other warm-up options available along the same principles if you wish to vary some of the exercises. This is not an issue as you may have problem areas that need more time. The message we are trying to put across is that the warm-up should be dynamic and prepare you for whatever session you maybe doing, as well as preparing you for the sessions which lie ahead.

Before every session you do, you need to perform a proper warm-up to raise the core temperature of your body. We call it Core Body Temperature or CBT warm-up. CBT warm-up with mobility should take between 10 and 15 minutes. You may want to take some time to loosen off pre warm-up, with bands and foam rollers.

James says:
"If you don't understand this warm-up and want to see actual examples then you can through our website **www.jameshaskell.com** or you can go to **YouTube** and search TheJamesHaskell – **www.youtube.com/thejameshaskell** to watch this specific warm-up and view others we have done."

You will be focusing on this warm-up for 12-15 minutes. I have given the example of doing each exercise for 1 minute. The idea is that you end up doing a couple of rounds of each exercise to take up the full 12-15 minutes. I have also detailed different variations of some of them for those working at a more advanced level.

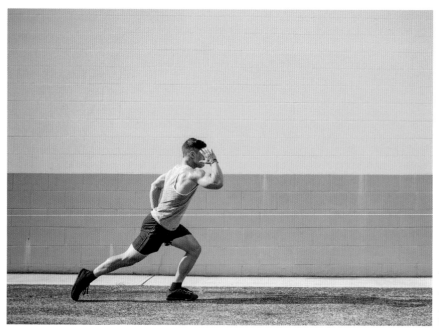

Picture Istock

W.1 - HIGH KNEES

Basic high knees can be performed while running in place or moving over a distance. Stand in place with your feet hip-width apart. Drive your right knee toward your chest and quickly place it back on the ground.

Follow immediately by driving your left knee toward your chest. Continue to alternate knees as quickly as you can.

Perform for 1 minute

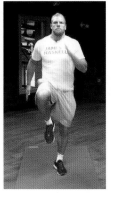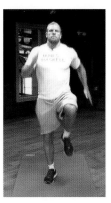

W.2 - HEEL FLICKS

The aim is to have a fast tempo. Use your arms to balance the body and drive the movement. Try to kick your bottom with the heels of your foot. It's not about the distance covered; it's more about the speed of movement. You should feel the stretch in your quads and hamstrings when doing this movement. Make sure you have a little forward lean as well.

Perform for 1 minute

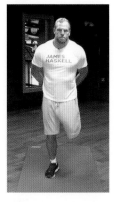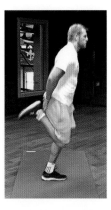

W.3 - STAR JUMPS

Perform by jumping to a position with the legs spread wide and the hands touching overhead and then return to a position with feet together, arms at sides. You can then repeat this movement dynamically.

Perform for 1 minute

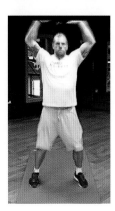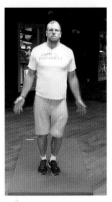

W.4 - LADDER DRILLS

Using cones or an SAQ ladder, start by facing down the ladder with both your feet together. You are going to then place one foot in each rung as you move through the ladder.

You are going to be doing this as quickly as possible. Its not an issue to be looking down at the ladder, as it's important you are accurate as well as quick. Once you reach one end you turn round and come back down the ladder.

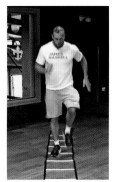
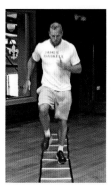

One foot in each rung

The next variation of this exercise is to face down the ladder once again. This time, however you are going to be placing two feet in each rung as you move up the ladder. Again you turn round quickly once you reach the end and come back down the ladder.

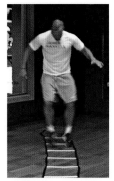
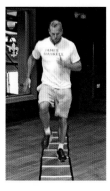

Two feet in each rung

Once you have cracked these two simple forward movements, you can then look to work on lateral movement. The easiest one of these is to start at the end of the ladder facing sideways so the ladder is lateral to you.

The first two you started front on. You are then going to laterally move down the ladder with two feet in each rung.

Once again when you reach the end, you turn round and come back the facing the same way but leading with the other leg.

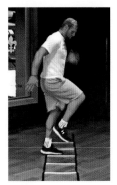
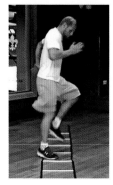

Laterals

James says:
"You can perform all three of these different variations in whatever way you fancy, continuously for the one minute."

30

James says:
"It's really important to focus on your arm movement and not just your feet when doing the ladder work. You are trying to be as dynamic as possible and your arms give you balance and speed. When you are starting off, looking down at the ladder is not a problem. However, the better you get, the more you want to avoid looking at the ladder. Rugby is all about watching what's happening in front of you. For example you wouldn't look down if a defender was coming at you and you wanted to use footwork."

Finally, if you find these first three really simple then we have given you some advanced options. These all come with there own videos on www.jameshaskell.com to help demo them.

The first is a lateral movement through the ladder where you start with the first rung in front of you, you then put two feet into that rung and quickly out again, as you move laterally in and out of the ladder.

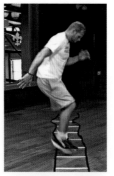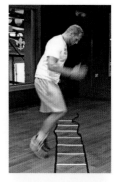

Laterals feet in and out

The next one is a plyometric jump step. You start in the same position as the last exercise, but with the inside foot in the rung and the other out, you then jump the inside out and the outside in. You do this while moving down the ladder. It's a really dynamic movement. You of course come back down the ladder when you reach the end.

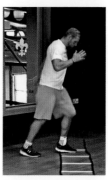

Plyo jump step lateral

The last advanced variation is the icky shuffle. You start to the side of the ladder with your inside foot in the first rung. You then take this foot out, onto the other side of the ladder and then bring the inside foot in to the next rung in the ladder and so forth as you move up the ladder. You then turn round at the end and come back down.

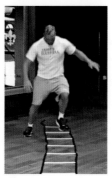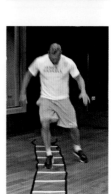

Icky shuffle

W.5 - WALK OUTS

Standing tall, bend over and touch the ground. Walk your hands out into a press-up position, or as far as you can go whilst maintaining good posture. Then walk your hands back in to where you started, until you fold back up to standing. You will feel the pull in your hamstrings.

This exercise is all about preparing your posterior chain, especially your hamstrings, which is particularly relevant to rugby players.

If your flexibility is poor then you will need to bend you knees as you curl down or curl back up. The ideal is straight legs, but technique is more important.

Perform for 1 minute

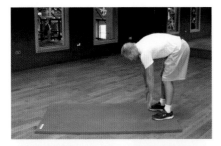
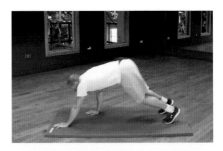
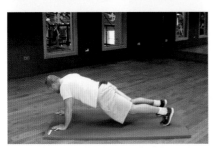
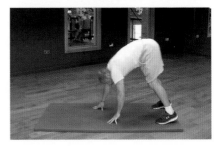

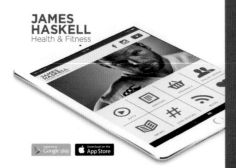

W.6 - LUNGE DRILLS

Forward lunges, reverse lunges, lateral lunges and curtsey lunges (lads: try to channel your inner polite girl, when doing these curtsey lunges. Ladies this should be easy for you).

Make sure you maintain good form and imagine you have a weight pulling you down through your middle when you lunge out, backwards and forwards.

You don't want to have your weight going forward when you lunge forward, your knee should never travel right over your foot. The leg goes out and then you go down feeling the stretch.

Repeat until you have done two full circuits

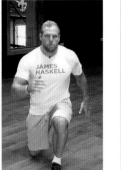

Forward   Reverse

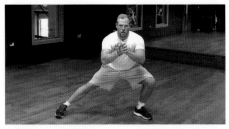

Lateral

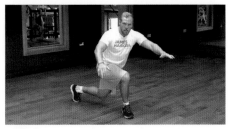

Curtsey

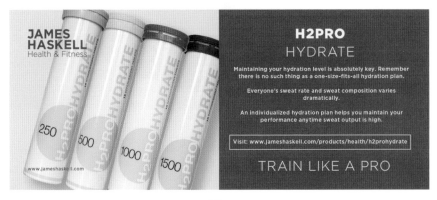

W.7 - KARAOKE DRILLS

These are very similar to side shuffles, but as you are shuffling side ways, one of your legs rotates in front and then behind.

You then come back the other way with the opposite leg going in front and then behind. When you are performing this exercise it is really important that you use your upper body as well as your lower body to help you rotate.

You need to turn your hips and arms to help you dynamically move. Don't just use your legs.

You want your body to be fluid when moving.

Perform for 1 minute

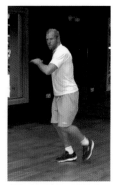
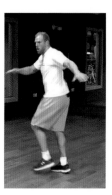

One foot in each rung

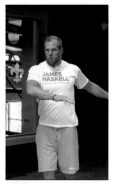
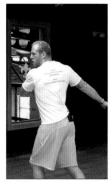

Arm technique breakdown

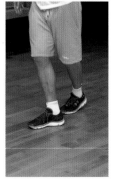

Leg technique breakdown

W.8 - LATERAL SIDE SHUFFLES

When performing the side shuffles it's really important that you have a slight bend in your knees, you keep your head up and your feet shoulder width apart. You will find yourself in a half squat position to make this movement really effective.

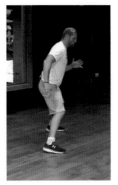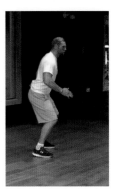

Make a lateral step to the right with your right foot. Bring your left foot to where your right foot was. As your left foot comes down, again move your right foot further right.

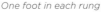
One foot in each rung

When you have covered enough distance (ideally 10 metres), switch back and go the other way. Remember to keep your feet parallel to the direction you are moving. The Shuffle exercise gets harder the further you go, and the quicker you move your feet.

Over time, increase the distance and speed you go. Bend your knees more and more through the shuffle to work your glutes more effectively.

You can progress this exercise using mini bands around your knees and ankles. They add tension and really switch on your glutes.

Perform for 1 minute

INSTRUCTION REVIEW

Make sure that you perform all the exercises above for a for a total of 10 minutes, going through each of them a couple of times for a full warm-up. As you become fitter and your technique improves, you can add in the variations suggested to increase the challenge. You can also look to extend this warm-up by a further 5 minutes, taking the total time to 15 minutes. You do this by repeating the exercises we have suggested with ever increasing speed and for longer than 1 minute.

STEP 3 HIIT CARDIO

HIIT sessions are a great way of getting a short, sharp, full-body conditioning blast. They also help you burn fat and stay in shape.

You will be working both aerobic and anaerobic training systems when undertaking a HIIT session and some of the other sessions that we cover off in this introduction guide.

Aerobic means "with oxygen," and Anaerobic means "without oxygen."

Aerobic training is any activity that stimulates your heart rate and increases your level of breathing. However not to the point where you can't sustain the activity. Anaerobic training will have you out of breath in just a few moments, like when you sprint. Both of these energy systems are used in rugby. During a game of rugby you are probably working continuously for between 45 seconds to around 3 minutes maximum. These are hard, intense patches of play, where you are required to execute different core skills, such as ball carrying, tackling, chasing kicks and getting on and off the floor.

It is not about straight line running. So your training has to match up with these levels of intensity. This is why something like HIIT (High Intensity Interval Training) is really important to add into your training plan.

Q&A

How often would you do this type of HIIT Cardio Training In-Season?

I would look to include a shortened version of this session once a week in my training as a general fitness top up. If I hadn't played or have had limited game time, then I would certainly look to use one of these sessions or a power endurance workout at the start of my week. To make it more suitable for in-season, I would bolt this session on after a weights workout at the start of my week, to give me the necessary cardio fitness top-up, which I will have missed out on from not playing.

How often would you do this type of training in pre-season?

This session, along with power endurance, would make up a key foundation to the conditioning block of my pre-season programme. Most pre-seasons are split into different sections, or phases. I would look to do one of these, or a power endurance type session twice a week, in the conditioning phase.

How often would you do this type of training in your down time/holidays?

This is great as a top-up during your down time. If you want to work out but don't want to spend hours in the gym, these HIIT workouts offer a perfect option. One or two times a week is fine. This is great for maintaining good body composition, weight and body fat management.

SESSION INSTRUCTIONS

You are working for 30 seconds on all these exercises and then resting for 90 seconds. Each one of these exercises is stand-alone. You perform 5 sets of an exercise before you move onto the next one.

H.1.1 - DUMBBELL THRUSTERS

Select two suitably weighted dumbbells. I suggest you don't start off by going too heavy.

Stand with your feet shoulder width apart. Have the dumbbells at shoulder level as shown in the pictures.

From a standing position you squat down, with your weight through your heels and your chest and head-up. You then power back-up, using your glutes and hamstrings, with a good hip drive.

When you nearly get back up to standing fully upright, you press the dumbbells above your head. Do this within the movement, which takes you to stand fully upright. The dumbbells then come back level with your shoulders and you repeat the whole movement again.

Perform 5 sets of 30 seconds of this before you move on with 90 seconds rest between sets.

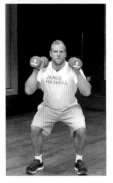
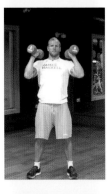

**Muscle Groups:
Quads, Glutes,
Hamstring,
Shoulders,
Lats, Traps**

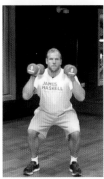

H.1.2 - ROWING MACHINE

Set the rower to medium
resistance. Row for 30 seconds
as hard as you can, but making
sure you are using the full range of
movement. Make sure you use your
legs as well as your upper body
when rowing.

*Perform 5 sets of 30 seconds of
this
before you move on with 90
seconds rest between sets.*

**Muscle Groups: Back, Lats,
Quads, Arms, Shoulders, Traps**

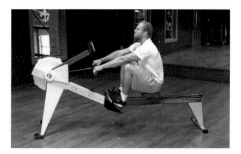

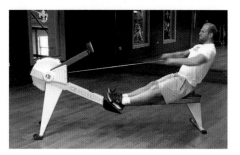

H.1.3 - WATTBIKE / SPIN BIKE

When preparing to do this bike
sprint, make sure that your seat
position is correct. Too many
people don't have this set correctly
and can cause themselves all sorts
of problems.

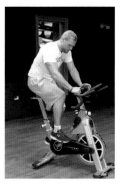

You need to have it high enough
so you get full leg extension. Also
make sure you get the right level of
resistance as you work. Your legs
should never just free spin on the
bike once you stop peddling, you
should always have some tension.
Be In control. Set this to medium
resistance. Sprint while staying
seated for 30 seconds.

*Perform 5 sets of 30 seconds of
this before you move on with 90
seconds rest between sets.*

**Muscle Groups: Legs, Lungs,
Hamstrings, Calves**

H.1.4 - MOUNTAIN CLIMBERS

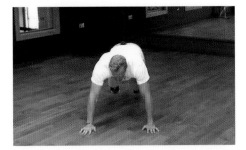

Start in a normal press-up position but with your feet wider apart than normal. You then bring one leg up to the outside of one of your arms. You should feel a stretch in your groin and hamstring. You keep the other leg straight.

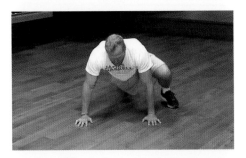

You then dynamically swap legs. So your other leg comes up towards your other hand, then the other leg goes back to where it came from and the first leg repeats the drill. You continue to do this alternating movement for the entire 30 seconds.

Alternatively, instead of having your feet come to the outside of your hands, you bring them up under your body as far as your flexibility will allow. Your legs will then move backwards and forwards in a straight line.

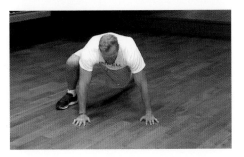

Perform 5 sets of 30 seconds of this before you move on with 90 seconds rest between sets.

Muscle Groups: Hip Flexors, Hamstrings, Glutes, Shoulders, Triceps, Forearms

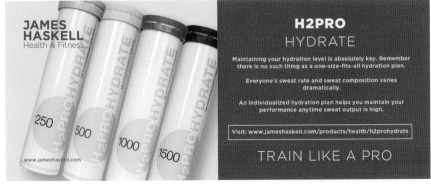

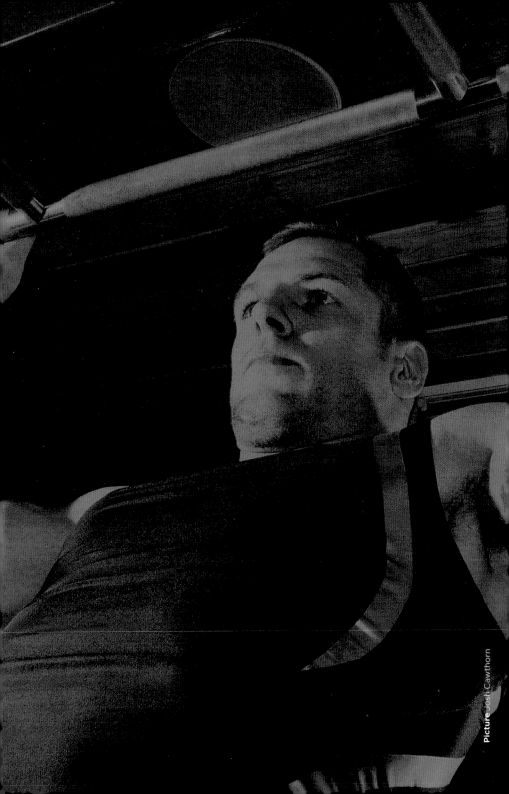

STEP 4 BODYWEIGHT TRAINING

James says:
"When I first joined Wasps I went straight into lifting weights, which in hindsight was the wrong way to do things in my mind. I wish I had spent some time working on my bodyweight strength; it would have helped me with performance and long-term gains."

Too many lads rush off to start doing bench press when they can't even do 20 press-ups. There is no point in leaping to lift weights if you can't even do 10 pull-ups of your own weight. So my recommendation to anyone who is looking to start training is take a while to focus on some bodyweight work. It 's simple, safe and will help you develop technique for other weighted lifts.

You will also see some really good changes with your body through this kind of workout. You can of course then progress to using suspension equipment like the TRX. Finally building to full weights.

Q&A

How often would you do this type of Bodyweight Training In-Season?

In season I would look to perform these sessions once a week, or more likely add these bodyweight exercises into my normal weights programme as complimentary exercises to my big lifts. If I was sore after a game then I may swap a weighted exercise for a bodyweight one, or first do a bodyweight session at the beginning of the week..

How often would you do this type of training in pre-season?

At the start of pre season when you are getting back into training, it is a good time to perform bodyweight work. Again like in season you can add it into to your weights sessions as complimentary exercises, or perform them as stand-alone sessions. If you are new to lifting then this is a great time to be doing it. I would suggest 1 or 2 sessions a week that either include bodyweight work or are complete bodyweight sessions.

How often would you do this type of training in your down time/ holidays?

This is the best type of training in your down time, it takes pressure off your joints but still works you hard. I make most of my sessions bodyweight focused, especially when on holiday and space is limited.
1 or 2 sessions per week.

UPPER BODY SESSION
STAND ALONE EXERCISES (NOT SUPER SET)

James says:
"If you struggle to perform any of these exercises, look into heavy-duty bands to take some of the weight. These work great on things like Pull-ups and Dips."

---

1 - PRESS UPS

Start in a usual press up position. You want to lower yourself down for a 3 count. Your hands should be placed shoulder width apart. As you lower down imagine pushing the floor together between your hands. You then push back up slowly.

- 3 sets of 10-20 reps

- Take between a 1 minute to 1 minute 30 second rest between sets

- Make sure you are working slowly on the eccentric and concentric phases. Aim for a 3, 2, 1 count eccentric and 1, 2 concentric

Muscle Groups: Chest, Shoulders, Biceps, Triceps, Abdominals

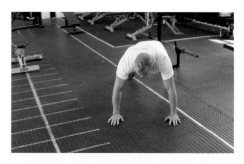

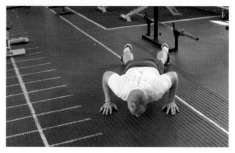

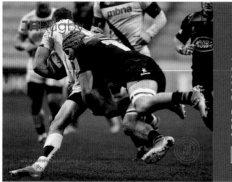

2 - TRICEP DIPS - BENCH OR NORMAL

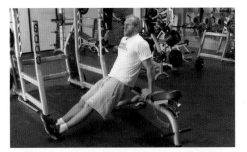

Find a bench that is strong enough to take your weight or some dip bars. Face away from the bench with your hands shoulder width, behind you on the edge. This exercise is for your triceps so you are taking the weight through the ball of your hands. You are lowering yourself down on a 3 count and pushing up on a 2 count. You have your feet out in front of you. The further they are away from you, the harder the exercise will become.

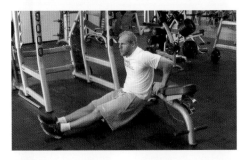

If you are using dip bars then you will stand between them, find a comfortable hand position and take your weight through the palms of your hands, raise yourself up and then lower yourself as low as you can go. Then repeat.

- 3 sets of 10-20 reps

- Take between a 1 minute to 1 minute 30 second rest between sets

- Make sure you are working slowly on the eccentric and concentric phases. Aim for a 3, 2, 1 count eccentric and 1, 2 concentric

Muscle Groups: Triceps, Biceps, Shoulders, Lats, Traps

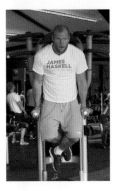
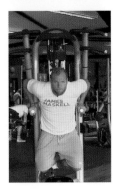

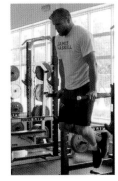
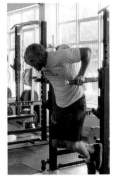

3 - CHINS UPS OR PULL UPS

To perform a Chin-up, which is the exercise shown in the picture, stand under either a straight bar or specialist Chin-up bar.

You need to use an underhand grip for a Chin-up.

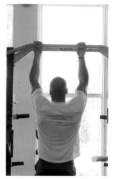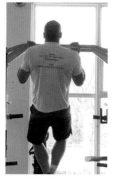

I find the best way to start is at the top of the movement. You either jump-up or step-up onto something, like a stepper to reach the bar. Pull yourself up, so your chin is level with the bar. You then lower yourself down to full extension for a 3-second count. You then pull yourself back up for a 2-second count.

Underhand grip Chin-up

Make sure you use the full range of movement at your disposal.

Pull-ups are exactly the same process and technique as detailed above, except for this exercise you are using an overhand grip, instead of an underhand grip.

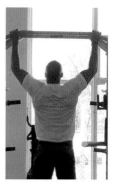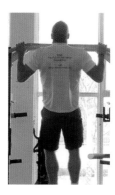

The last and easiest alternative to either a Chin-ups or a Pull-ups is the neutral grip Chin-up. Please see the last photograph for more detail. The method for neutral grip is the same as a Chin-up, except you are using a neutral grip.

Overhand Pull-up

- 3 sets of 8 - 15 reps
- Take between a 1 minute to 1 minute 30 second rest between sets
- Make sure you are working slowly on the eccentric and concentric phases. Aim for a 3, 2, 1 count eccentric and 1, 2 concentric

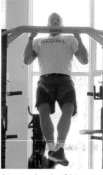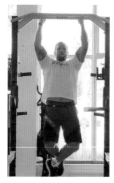

Muscle Groups: Biceps, Shoulders, Back, Lats, Traps, Forearms, Grip

Neutral grip Chin-up

44

STEP 5 RESISTANCE TRAINING

Within this package I have talked about the benefits of resistance training for a rugby player. If you want to make any sort of strength, size or power gains then you are going to need to lift weights. As this package is all about an "Introduction to Rugby fitness" I have provided only a lower body workout.

The reasons behind this are as follows: To be a rugby player, leg drive, power and strength are integral. Too many players spend their time working on upper body sessions. Don't get me wrong, upper body strength is important, however I want to give you a taste of a really good leg session, which I have done.

When we produce a package just focussed on getting big for rugby, we will cover the upper body. If you want try something now, visit our Youtube channel under www.youtube.com/thejameshaskell to see some specific upper body workouts.

If you are looking to put on size and build strength, then you need to lift weights.
There is a lot of confusion out there over what kind of weightlifting you need to do. The answer is you need to be doing Hypertrophy Training: This is 'Time Under Tension' work focussed on a rep range of between 8 and 12 reps.

You need to perform all these lifts with good control over the concentric and eccentric ranges. Or to put it more simply, the raising and lowering of the weight needs to be done with a slowness to really activate the muscle. For example if you did bench press (not a great exercise for rugby players) you would unrack the bar and lower it down for a count of 3, 2, 1. Then push up over a count of 1, 2. The amount you lift should be based on how well you can perform the movement, whilst maintaining good control and form. For example, if you are doing 10 reps and the last 2 are a real struggle, then that is the perfect weight. Don't become obsessed with trying to lift too much at the start. We will cover specific strength training in another package.

Q&A

How often would you do this type of Resistance Training In-Season?
In season I would look to perform a maximum of three weights sessions per week. These would be split between one lower body, one upper body and one power session. If I only have time for one then I would always go for lower body. I always front load these sessions to the beginning of the week, with power being towards the end of the week. You don't want to be sore to play!

How often would you do this type of training in pre-season?
Pre-season is where you get most of your size and strength gains. You would be looking to do anywhere between four to five weight sessions a week. However, like all pre-seasons it depends what phase you are in and what your goals are. Size building is mainly done in the first phase.

How often would you do this type of training in your down time/holidays?
In my down time I like to keep things pretty relaxed, but I would certainly do two short weight sessions every week to keep things ticking over. These would not be about lifting huge weights, but rather hypertrophy training, bodyweight work or fun circuits.

LEG SESSION
SET 1 - STAND-ALONE

R.4.1.1 - BARBELL BACK SQUAT

Place a barbell across your shoulders. Feet shoulder width apart. Keeping your chest up and back straight, squat back, taking all the weight through your heels. The aim is to retain your form to just below parallel. You then focus on hip drive to push you back up to standing. The speed you should squat on the downward part is a three count. I.e. 3, 2, 1, pause at the bottom for 1 second then power back up. Make sure that you only go to the depth that you can maintain form. You will hear about depth being key, but if you can't keep your form then you can't go to that depth. It's something to build towards.

- Perform four sets of 10 – 12 reps before you move on.

- Rest or between 1 minute to 1 minute 30 seconds between each set

- Alternative exercise – Bodyweight Squat

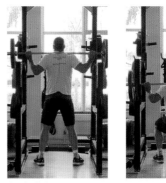

Barbell Squat

Muscle Groups:
Quads, Hamstrings, Glutes, Abductors, Adductors, Abdominals, Lower Back

SET 2 - SUPER SET

R.4.2.1 - A. ROMANIAN DEAD LIFT

Put a barbell in front of you on the ground and grab it using a pronated (palms facing down) grip that is a little wider than shoulder width. Bend the knees slightly and keep the shins vertical, hips back and back straight. This will be your starting position. Keeping your back and arms completely straight at all times, use your hips to lift the bar as you exhale. The movement should not be fast but steady and under control.

Once you are standing completely straight up, lower the bar by pushing the hips back, only slightly bending the knees. You should feel all the tension through your hamstrings as you lower the bar. Keep your head up. When you have reached the depth you are comfortable with, use a good hip drive to take the bar back-up to the starting position, tensing your glutes as you do.

- Perform one set of 10 reps of this, before moving straight onto the Dumbbell Bulgarian Lunge. Once completed, rest for between 1 minute to 1 minute 30 seconds. That is one complete Superset. Perform three Supersets in total

- Alternative exercise – Swiss Ball Hamstring Curls

Muscle Groups: Hamstrings, Glutes, Lower Back, Traps and Shoulders, Abdominal

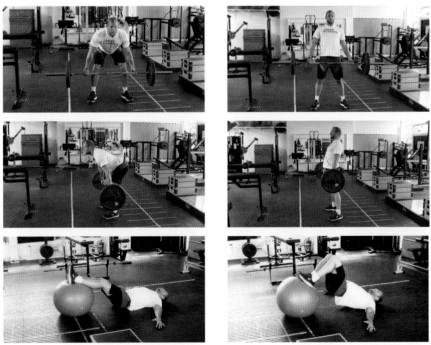

Alternate - Swiss Ball Hamstring Curls

R.4.2.2 - B. DUMBBELL BULGARIAN SPLIT SQUAT

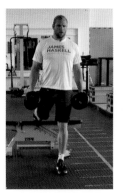
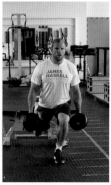

Stand with your back facing a gym bench, step box or something off the ground. Place a foot on the box behind you and step forward with the other leg, with the dumbbells in each hand. I suggest you adopt a lighter weight than you might otherwise use, as you need to keep your balance and form. Lunge onto the front leg, maintaining a strong posture. Go as low as you can, allowing for what your flexibility or strength permits. Imagine you have a piece of string running down your middle and you are trying to go straight down, not forward. Then drive back-up, keeping the weight through the heel of the outstretched foot.

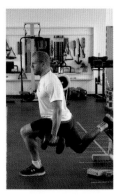
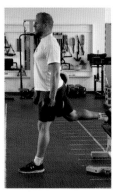

- Perform 8 reps of this exercise. You then rest for between 1 minute to 1 minute 30 seconds. As this is a Super set, you then go back to Romanian Deadlift. You perform three Supersets in total

The alternative – Bodyweight Lunge Walk

PERFORM THREE SETS OF A SUPER SET IN TOTAL

Muscle Groups:
Quads, Hamstrings, Abductors, Abdominals, Adductors, Glutes

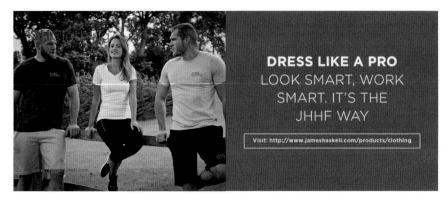

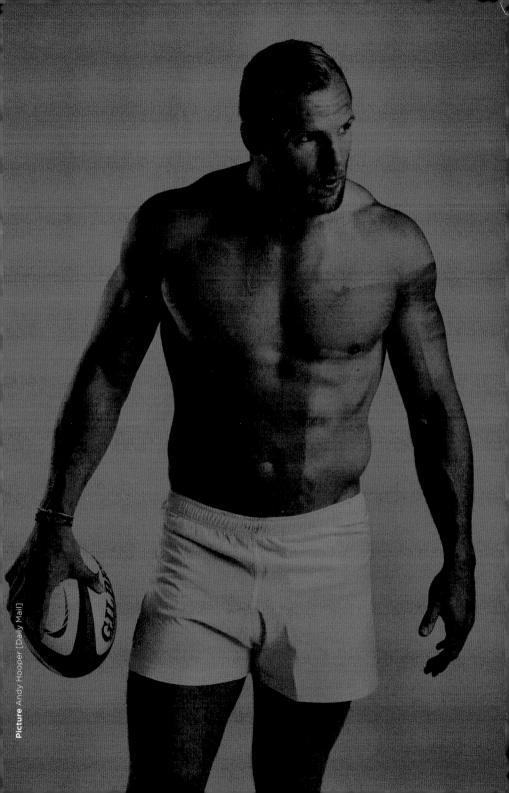

SET 3 - SUPER SET

R.4.3.1 - A. SEATED LEG EXTENSION

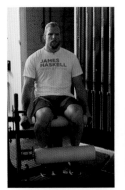
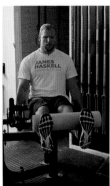

For this exercise you will need to use a leg extension machine. First choose your weight and sit on the machine with your legs under the pad (feet pointed forward) and the hands holding the sidebars. This will be your starting position. Make sure that your legs form a 90-degree angle between the lower and upper leg. If the angle is less than 90-degrees then that means the knee is over the toes, which in turn creates undue stress at the knee joint. Using your quadriceps, extend your legs to the maximum as you exhale.

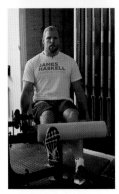

Ensure the rest of the body remains stationary on the seat. The raising phase should be a 3 count. Then pause for 5 seconds on the contracted position at the top, lower for a three count. An alternative to doing both leg-up and down's is to use two legs to take the bar-up and then one leg to slowly lower it back down. This intensifies the exercise.

You can alternate exercise and do single legs rather than double

- Perform one set of 10 reps. Then move straight onto the Glute Bridge. You then rest for between 1 minute to 1 minute 30 seconds. You are completing three Super sets in total

Muscle Group: Quads

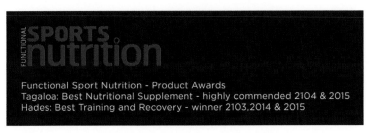

R.4.3.2 - B. GLUTE BRIDGE

Begin seated on the ground with a bench directly behind you. You can do this with a barbell across your lap, or if you are starting out you can have a loaded barbell over your legs. If you decide to weight these, then you will need to rest the bar on a pad across your lap. I would recommend doing these bodyweight to start. The focus of this movement is to drive your hips up, and take your weight through your feet. It's really important you get the full extension in your hips. You tense your glutes at the top. The other option is to do this exercise with your back on a bench. The start position if very simple. You have your feet on the floor and your shoulder on the bench. You then have a bend in the middle.

You begin the movement by driving through your feet, extending your hips vertically up, tensing your glutes at the top of the movement. Hold for 3 seconds. When doing this exercise you should feel tension in your hamstring but mainly your glutes. Your weight should be supported by your shoulder blades and your feet. Extend as far as possible, then reverse the motion to return to the starting position. This is the same technique as you would use if using the Swiss Ball, if you don't have a bench to hand.

- Repetitions – perform one set of 10 reps. Then rest for between 1 minute to 1 minute 30 seconds between Super sets. Starting back on seated leg extensions. You are performing 3 Super sets in total

The alternative – Bodyweight Glute Bridge on floor with mini band between knees

Muscle Groups: Hamstring, Glutes, Calves, Hip Flexors

Using a bench

Alternative - on the floor

Alternative - using an exercise ball

SET 4 - SUPER SET

R.4.4.1 - A. GLUTE HAM RAISE

Begin by adjusting the equipment to fit your body. Place your feet against the footplate in between the rollers as you lie facedown. Your knees should be just behind the pad. Start from the bottom of the movement. Keep your back slightly arched as you begin the movement by flexing your knees. You should be pulling yourself up using your hamstrings and glutes.

By the mid-point when you become horizontal, you should be tensing your glutes. Drive your toes into the footplate as you do so. Keep your upper body straight and head up; continue until your body is upright. Return to the starting position, keeping your descent under control. I suggest if you are starting out you only go to horizontal, making sure your hamstring and glutes take the tension. You then hold at this level for a couple of seconds and return to the start position. Do not over arch your back, or use your back to pull you up. Make sure you do this movement with a slow and controlled motion.

An alternative to this is to use a Swiss Ball. You lay on the floor with your heels on the ball. Keeping your core on and your hips up, drag the ball into your bottom then slowly let it roll away. Whilst performing this exercise you should feel this in your hamstrings and glutes the entire time.

- Perform one set of 10 reps before moving straight onto Calf Raise. You are performing Three Super sets in total
- Alternative exercise – Hamstring Ball Pulls using a Swiss Ball

Muscle Groups: Hamstrings, Glutes, Lower Back

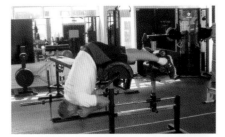
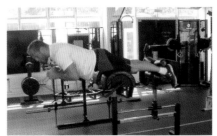

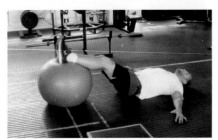
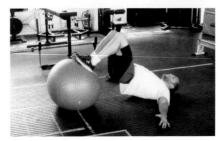

Alternative - using a Swiss Ball

R.4.4.2 - B. STANDING CALF RAISE

You can do this on the floor or you can do this on a raised block. Your gym may have a specific calf raise machine you can use as well, either with or without weight. It all depends what level you are at, the principle movement of this exercise is the same whether you are using a machine or just body weight on a raised block. Standing feet slightly apart, raise your heels as you breathe out by extending your ankles as high as possible and flexing your calf. Ensure the knee is kept stationary at all times. There should be no bending at any time. Hold the contracted position for a second before you start to go back down. Go back slowly to the starting position. As you breathe in lower your heels as you bend the ankles, until your calves are stretched.

- Repetitions – perform one set of 10 reps. Then rest for between 1 minute to 1 minute 30 seconds. Go back to Glute Ham Raise. You are performing three Super sets in total

Muscle Group: Calves

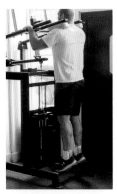
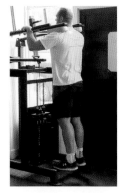

Feet movement:

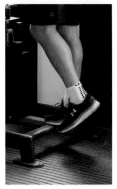
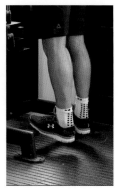

Feet movement - single leg raise

Feet movement - double leg raise

The other way of performing this exercise, if you don't have access to a special calf raise machine, is to use a raised box on the floor.

You can see what a raised box looks like in the images to the right. You will find these type of boxes in most gyms.

Please note, the technique required for performing the exercise on a raised box is the same technique required to perform the exercise on an actual calf raise machine.

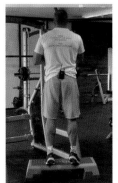
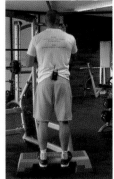

Stepper Box

STEP 6 POWER ENDURANCE

It is not practical to play contact rugby every day for many reasons; injury and fatigue being the main ones. You would be in no shape to perform when it came to game day. The power endurance sessions that I describe in this plan are there to try and replicate some of the game movements and also to condition the body for the rigours of playing rugby. The exercises we use in these sessions are very functional and will keep you moving. They will also tire your entire body just like rugby does.

Unlike the HIIT sessions these are much harder and would be stand alone sessions.

There are both gym based and outdoor versions, which you can apply to your training. You can often put the two together to form an indoor and outdoor session.

On the next page, I am going to give you an example of an outdoor version we would do in our professional training programme.

Q&A

How often would you do this type of Power Endurance Training In-Season?
I would look to include a shortened version of this session once a week in my training as a top-up if I felt I needed it. This would mainly be at the beginning or middle of the season. If I hadn't played or had limited game time, then I would certainly look to perform one of these sessions. To make it more suitable for in-season I would bolt this session on after a weights workout at the beginning of the week, or combine it with some running fitness. I would reduce the reps and group the exercises into a circuit, as if it was a small top-up session.

How often would you do this type of training in pre-season?
This session along with HIIT training would make up a key foundation to the conditioning block of my pre-season programme. Most pre-seasons are split into different sections, or phases. I would look to do one of these or a HIIT type session twice a week. I would do one block of this combined with running as part of a pre-season fitness sessions. For example, you may have four blocks of different types of conditioning in one session selecting two exercises from power endurance/running. For example - power endurance, running, power endurance, running. Obviously with the appropriate rest in between sets. The session I am suggesting could look like this: you would have a block of power endurance, followed by running, then more power endurance and finally end with running. Obviously within this session you would have the appropriate rest, number of sets and so forth. The session may take 45 - 55 minutes in total to complete. This includes warm-up and rest.

How often would you do this type of training in your down time/holidays?
These sessions are quite tough for your down-time but are great workouts. If you are looking to rest from running, they will still give you a good conditioning hit. I would look at performing one of these tougher sessions only once a week in my down time. If I am honest I would rather do one of these harder sessions than loads of little conditioning blocks. When the weather is good, I love to get the prowlers out, sleds, tyres and sledgehammers. It's fun, hard and you really feel like you've worked. These sessions are best done with a training partner.

POWER ENDURANCE SESSION - CIRCUIT

1 - SLED OR PROWLER PUSH

Choose either method one or method two.
You are working for 20 seconds per exercise.

With Sled/Prowler: The focus of this exercise is to keep a good long stride length as you push the sled. Make sure you keep your back flat and your head up as you drive the sled for 15 metres as hard as you can. Then after 15 metres turn it around and push it back again, as fast as you can. Obviously you keep continuously pushing the sled for the allotted 20 second work time.

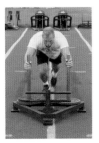

Without Sled/Prowler – Partner method:
Alternative to a sledge push is a partner resisted leg drive. Ask your partner to stand in front of you with their hands on your shoulders. They need to be able to brace themselves to take the force. You set yourself in a good running position leaning well forward, so your partner is taking some of your weight. You then run forward while your partner resists you for the 15 metres or however far you push your partner in the 20 second work time. You can get them to vary the level of resistance. However for this to be effective you do need some moderate resistance.

If you choose Method One, you are working for 20 seconds, resting for 5 to 10 seconds, before you move onto the next exercise.

Method Two, you are working for 20 seconds then resting for 10 seconds, repeating the same exercise five times in total. Rest for 1 minute 30 seconds before moving onto the next exercise.

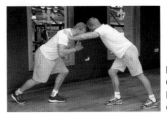

**Muscle Groups:
Quads, Calves,
Hamstrings,
Glutes**

2 - TYRE FLIPS

This exercise can be performed with a tyre (Method One) or without (Method Two). Either way, you will flip the item one way, then run round to the other side and flip it back. So the tyre/item should always stay where it is.

With Tyre: For this exercise technique is really important. Make sure you are using your legs to drive up the tyre. Find one that you can flip that isn't so heavy you lose your form.

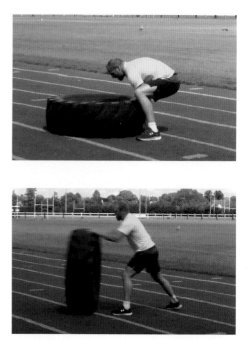

Key pointers of this are to keep your chest and head up. Make sure you take the weight through your heels. Use a good hip drive to get the tyre up. The deadlift technique is very similar to this and please note the same safety points apply. So flip one way. Then run around the tyre and flip it the other way, and so on.

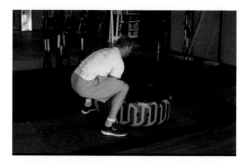

No Tyre – Tackle bag option: If you don't have a tyre, you can use a heavy full size tackle bag/tackle tube. You flip the heavy tackle bag end on using the same principles as detailed above.

If you choose Method One you are working for 20 seconds, resting for between 5 to 10 seconds, before moving onto the next exercise.

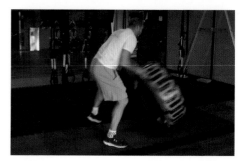

Method Two, you are working for 20 seconds, then resting for 10 seconds before repeating the same exercise five times in total. Rest for 1 minute 30 seconds before moving onto the next exercise.

Muscle Groups: Quads, Glutes, Shoulders, Biceps, Lower Back, Upper Back, Forearms and Abdominals

3 - LIZARD CRAWL (AKA BEAR CRAWL)

The idea of this exercise is to crawl forward using your hands and toes. You are not crawling on your knees. You need to keep your back flat and your bum down. You want to be dynamic and fast with this movement.

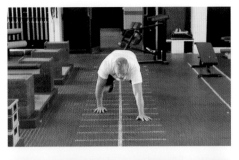

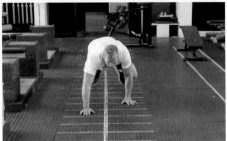

Crawl as far as you can in the 20 seconds. If you have limited space, then reach the end and crawl back. To make this harder you can crawl backwards.

If you choose Method One you are working for 20 seconds, resting for 5 to 10 seconds, before moving onto the next exercise.

Method Two, you are working for 20 seconds then resting for 10 seconds. Repeat the same exercise five times in total. Rest for 1 minute 30 seconds before moving onto the next exercise.

Muscle Groups: Shoulders, Quads, Hamstrings, Glutes, Abdominals, Abductors, Adductors, Calves

---

4 - MEDICINE BALL SLAM

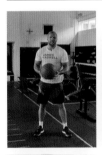
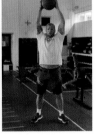
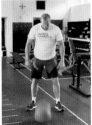

Muscle Groups: Shoulders, Lats, Upper Back, Triceps, Abdominals

Make sure you get a suitable weighted ball. The idea is to start holding the ball near to your chest. You then raise the ball above your head, making sure you extend up as far as possible. You then slam the ball into the ground as hard and fast as possible. The ball should bounce back up. If it doesn't then you just have to pick it off the floor. Whether you catch it or not, repeat the movement for 20 seconds. Make sure you use your full range of movement.

If you choose Method One you are working for 20 seconds, resting for 5 to 10 seconds, before moving onto the next exercise.

Method Two, you are working for 20 seconds, then resting for 10 seconds. Repeat the same exercise five times in total. Rest for 1 minute 30 seconds before moving onto the next exercise.

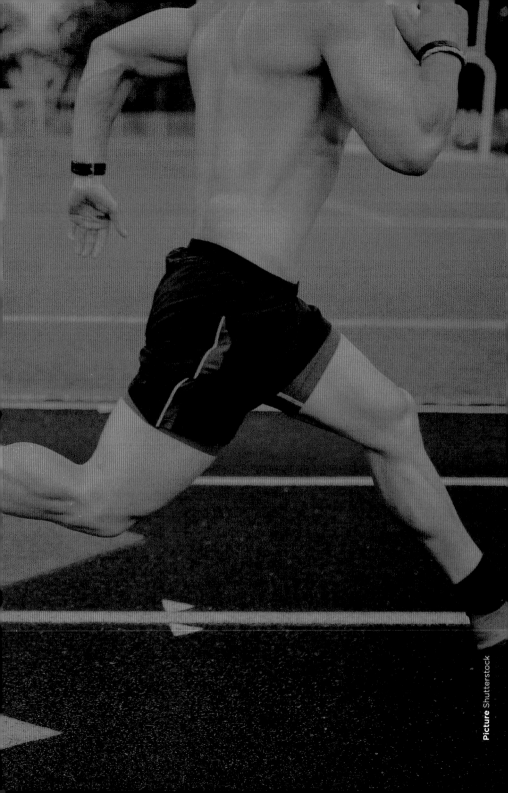

STEP 7 RUNNING SESSION

So far we have looked at a number of areas of conditioning and training. They all have different benefits for your rugby training and physical development. However one of the most important areas of conditioning to be a rugby player is the development of a running base.

Establishing a good running base can be achieved in various ways. Conditioners and trainers often talk about building a long distance endurance base for players, but my view is slightly different. Yes, you certainly need to have an endurance base to sustain your intensity throughout a game; but you are a rugby player, not a marathon runner. Therefore you very rarely work for any longer than three to four minutes maximum at one time during a game. As such, building power and endurance you can sustain at high intensities across a shorter time period, is far more important than being able to run continuously for an hour.

James says:
"After twelve years of playing professional rugby I've have developed an endurance which never diminishes, even if I have four weeks off. This is great but to maintain it I still have to put the work in and top myself up with running sessions. I would favour other sessions in the off-season over running, because of the impact it has on your joints. Add some shuttles into the mix, as well as HIIT and Power endurance. It is important to never get complacent with your routine. You need to constantly improve and diversify."

Q&A

How often would you do this type of Running Training In-Season?
At the start of the season I would look to top up my running fitness once a week. These would be a short sharp sessions bolted on after rugby training during the first part of the week. As the season progresses and I play more rugby, I would reduce this down to as and when I felt I needed it. Or if I had limited game time on the weekend, or no match at all, I would also do a running session to make sure I got a cardio and running top up.

How often would you do this type of training in pre-season?
I look to do two or three sessions a week of some sort of running conditioning, whether that is from rugby sessions, or specific conditioning sessions as detailed below. Your fitness coach might want you to do more or less running, as there are many views as to what works best. Some feel you should do less running but get most of your fitness from actual games. I feel you need some sort of base before you play. However the first game of the season is always horrific, no matter what you have done, so don't be surprised.

How often do you do this type of training in your down time/holidays?
I would normally not focus too much on running fitness until the last week of my holiday, where I would perhaps perform one or two sharp sessions. I may add some shuttle running into one of my power endurance or HIIT circuits to make sure you have some running in your legs and to change things up.

You can bolt running sessions on the end of most of your other forms of training if you do not have time for exclusive running sessions.

SESSION 1 - ON FIELD RUNNING SESSION

Muscle Groups worked on: Lungs, Legs, Upper Body
Skills: Running, Agility

R.S.1 - 15-15'S

Start standing on the try line:
- Sprint to far 22-metre line in 15 seconds
- 15 seconds rest
- Sprint back to far try line again in 15 seconds
- 10 sets of this – should take 6 minutes in total

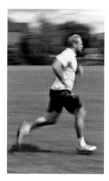

You are covering a total distance of about 72 metres in the 15 seconds. The idea of this session is to arrive at the line on the count of fifteen or just before it, i.e. 13, 14 seconds. This is an endurance session so you need to be pushing yourself. Equally don't go mental and become unable to finish it. If you are making the line too easily, or not at all then you can either increase or decrease the distance you are running in the 15 seconds. If you are doing sets of 10 and falling short on rep 8, 9, 10 it's not the end of the world. If you are missing it from the start then you need to reduce it. Equally if you are smashing it then you need to push yourself and increase the distance.

After 10 reps of this, rest for 2 minutes, then move onto Part Two - Down and Ups

Below is an example of some of the distances that you want to be getting to, based on Yoyo test levels.

Your target distance is:
86m (level 18 of the yoyo test)
89m (level 19 of the yoyo test)
91m (level 20 of the yoyo test)

Rest 2 minutes and move onto part 2 of the fitness session

What is a yoyo test?
(The Yoyo test is something we use to work out our level of base fitness at the beginning of the season, and throughout. You can find out more online about this system of measurement by Googling yoyo test). Take it from me - it is not fun!

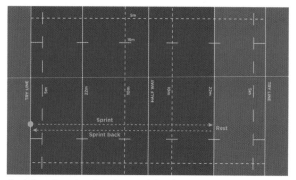

Part One Running Session explained

60

PART 2

R.S.2 - DOWN AND UPS

Start on the try line on your stomach. Get up and run to the 5-metre line, perform a down and up (chest to the floor), turn around sprint back to the try line and perform a down and up.

- Repetitions - 10 reps is one set. Repeat two sets of 10 reps completely through in total
- Rest for 1 minute between sets
- The aim to complete each set in under 30 seconds

Rest 2 minutes
Then repeat part 1 (the running session) again

Rest 2 minutes
Then repeat part 2 (the down & ups session) again

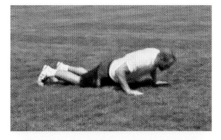 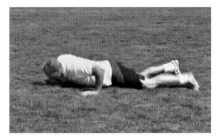

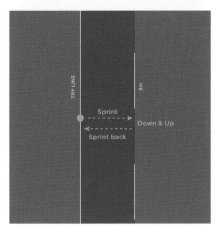

STEP 8 RUGBY-SPECIFIC CONDITIONING

You can't beat playing in an actual rugby match to attain the proper level of fitness. However you need to put some of your core skills under pressure during training in order to help develop them. For this session to work you will need some equipment or a partner. You can of course do a lot of this live, i.e. one on one with a teammate full contact if you wish.

James says:
"The example session I am going to give you focuses on tackle technique and competing for the ball."

Equipment you need:
* Big hit tackle pad (Rhino Rugby supply these)
* Tackle shield
* Partner
* Rugby ball

Q&A

How often would you do this type of Rugby Conditioning Training In-Season?
At the start of the season I would look to top up my conditioning once a week. This would either be with a straight running session, or a rugby-specific fitness workout. These would be short sharp sessions at the beginning of the week. As the season progresses and I play more rugby, I would reduce this down to when I felt I needed it, or when I have had limited or no game time at all. I would do this type of conditioning in the weeks where we didn't have a game, to keep myself fit and rugby focused. It is also fun to do as opposed to standard conditioning.

How often would you do this type of training in pre-season?
One or two sessions a week of some sort of rugby specific conditioning, whether that is something as simple as bag hits and running, or something more complicated as detailed below.

How often would you do this type of training in your down time/holidays?
Never really, I would try to get a rugby ball in my hands in my down time to practice my skills, but in terms of this type of conditioning it is not really practical.

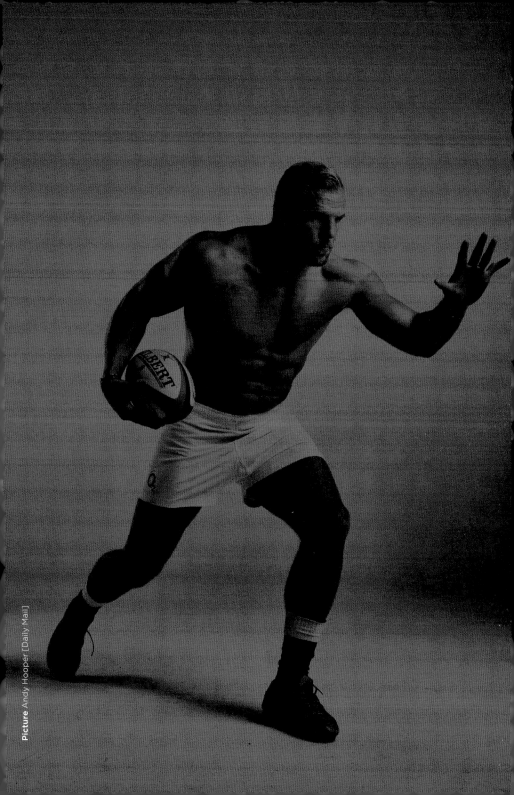

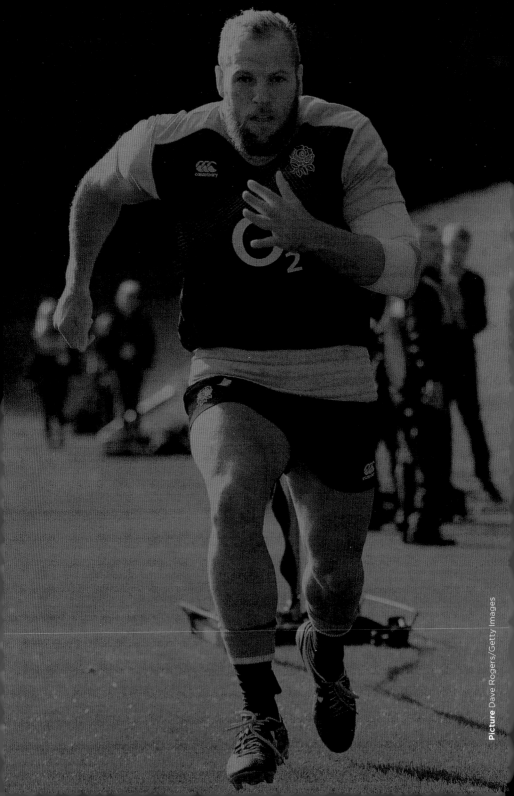

SESSION 1 - TACKLE PAD CONDITIONING

Skills: Tackling, Competing for the ball, Running

Start on your chest on the try line. The tackle pad is standing up on the 5-metre line. On the whistle or go, you run out and make a low tackle on the pad. Bounce to your feet straight away and run to the 22-metre line. You turn on the line and run back to the try line, where you perform a down and up. (Chest to the ground).

By this time your partner has placed a ball on the opposite side of the tackle pad you hit on the first movement. He is standing in front of the ball, holding a tackle shield. You get back to your feet and run in to compete for the ball. The bag acts as the tackled player. As you do this, your partner applies pressure, trying to stop you getting the ball. Once you have pulled the ball off the floor, you run to the 22-metre line. Walk back and rest on the try line.

- 6 reps of this drill is a Set
- Rest for 1 minute between each rep (If you are working with a team mate, then alternate with your partner if you want. I.e. you go and then he goes. So you are both getting one-to-one rest. When he reaches the 22-metre line, he walks back into place. Once there, then you go again)
- Perform 2 sets
- Rest for 2 minutes between the sets.

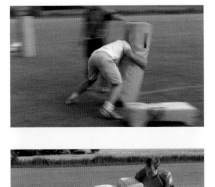

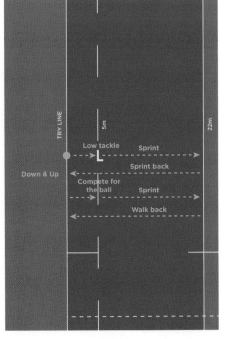

SESSION 2 - FOOTWORK, EVASION AND CONTACT SKILLS CONDITIONING

This is a stand-alone session, which should only be done on conditioning days. It's a tough session and not to be undertaken close to an actual game day. You can take one drill and add it into another session, if you don't want to do the full amount in one go.

The idea behind this session is to work on your ball carrying, passing and footwork.

To perform this session you will need the following items of equipment:
• Use of marked-out rugby field or a suitable area
• Three players
• Rugby ball
• 2 x tackle shields
• Stop watch
• Whistle

DRILL INSTRUCTIONS

Use the 10-metre to 22-metre lines as your channel length and work within the 15-metre line and the touch line as your channel width. You will need some space in which to perform but not too much. For the third part of the drill you will need to reduce the grid down width wise, to the 5-metre line and the touch line. So you are working the same length, 10-metre to 22-metre line, but much narrower to put your passing skills under pressure.

See Drill 1 on following page

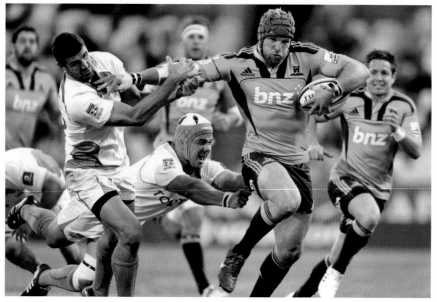

Picture Associated Press Images

66

DRILL 1

Position one player in the middle of the "marked" area as detailed above. The player with the ball needs to stand just outside the area. The third player (the attacking player) is on the 10-metre line, facing down the field.

Although this is a non-contact session, you are working hard for 30 seconds in this drill.

On the go call or whistle, the player who is outside the designated grid (who is also the time-keeper) either kicks or passes the ball to the player standing on the 10-metre line, who is facing down the field. (The player outside the grid can vary which side he stands and how far or close he is to the attacking player without the ball.) The attacking player then catches the ball and tries his best to beat the player in the middle of the grid with footwork and speed. The defender moves as soon as the ball is passed.

There must be no contact but the defending player does need to try to stop the attacking player with a firm touch/grasp. If the attacking player fails to beat the defender out right, then the defender should allow him through, so the drill can continue. If he gets a good grab on the player, he can hold him for a couple of seconds and then let him go. This will also be a fitness session for the defender as he needs to test the attacking player.

However if the attacking player manages to evade the defender, he then sprints all the way through to the 22-metre line. Once the player reaches the 22-metre line, he turns straight round and tries to beat the defender again. He repeats this process as many times as he can for 30 seconds. The defender can vary how much space he allows the attacking player. Make sure you create different scenarios for them.

The attacking and defending player

in the grid are both working for 30 seconds. Then they rest for 20 seconds. Once they have rested, all three players rotate round. You keep doing this until each player has attacked four times.

Rest for two minutes..

PHASE 1

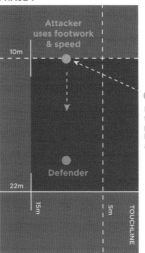

PHASE 2

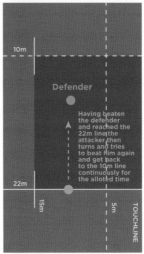

DRILL 2

You have one attacker, who again starts on the 10-metre line. This time the other two players standing in the grid are holding tackle shields with a gap between them. One of the bag holders holds a ball in a free hand.

On the whistle, the player with the ball throws the ball to the attacker. He can vary how he throws it to him; high, low, direct or even rolls it on the floor. The attacker gets the balls and then runs at the two defenders with the bag. The idea is he has to take contact this time. So as soon as the attacker catches the ball, the defenders can move up to get him and close down his space.

Once the attacker takes contact, the idea is for him to use his leg drive, bump and hand-off to get through the bags. The bags need to put up some resistance but ultimately must let the attacker through.

Once through the defenders, the attacker then sprints all the way through to the 22-metre line. As with the first exercise, he turns and repeats the same drill on the way back. The defenders need to vary how much space they give the attacker and how much space they give the attacker and how much gap they give the player to get through with the bags. You want to make sure you create scenarios, so he can utilise different techniques. Like bumping a player off, head down into low space or a hand off, if you have more time.

He works for 30 seconds and then swaps round as in part one. The drill is over once each player has attacked four times.

Rest for two minutes

PHASE 1

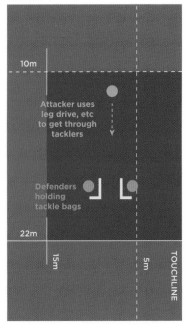

PHASE 2

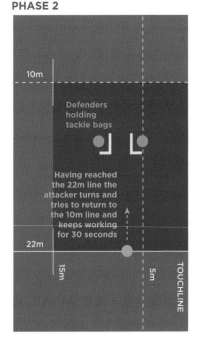

DRILL 3

Important instruction - reduce the grid down width wise, to the 5-metre line and the touch line. So you are working the same length, 10-metre to 22-metre line, but much narrower to put your passing skills under pressure. For this last drill you are working in pairs but this time with one defender and two attackers. For this drill there are two players on the 10- metre line, one of them has the ball. The defender is not using a tackle bag.

On the whistle, the player with the ball attacks the defender. He tries to beat him and either offloads to his supporting player or passes before contact. The defender is just grabbing, he is not tackling. Because of the reduced space this will really put your skills under pressure. The defender has, like in the first two parts of the drill, a really important role to play. He needs to either pressurise the attacker with the ball forcing an offload, or back off allowing a pass before contact.

If he grabs the player with the ball, as in Drill 1, he should allow the play to continue and the player to offload instead of a pass before contact.

The second player who caught the ball then sprints to the 22-metre line, he then turns round and this time as he still has the ball, he becomes the lead attacker. He tries to beat the defender and either offloads once grabbed or, ideally, makes a pass before contact. It is up to him to make the decision. It is a competition to get the ball away first.

The pair of attackers are working for 20 seconds. They rest for 10 seconds. Then one of the two attacking players becomes the defender. You do this until each player has defended twice.

NOTE THE CHANGE IN THE WORK TIME.

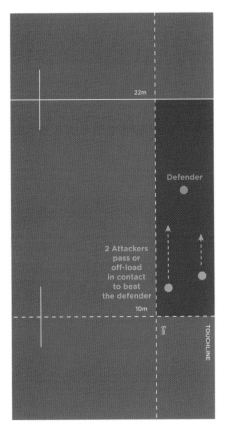

STEP 9 RUGBY CORE SKILL DRILLS
- COMPETING FOR THE BALL

James says:
"There are hundreds of drills out there to help you improve core skills, from simple passing, to full on tackle technique. As previously mentioned, you need to be taking ten minutes every day to practice these core skills after training. I have loads of specific drills I like to use to help me develop each area of my game."

The example I am giving is to focus on your breakdown steal work.

Q&A

How often would you do this type of Training In-Season?
I spend ten minutes every day after my rugby sessions working on one of my core skills. I focus on my strengths and work on my weaknesses in equal measure. I do more of the contact based work at the start of the week.

How often would you do this type of training in pre-season?
After every skill session or rugby session I work on my core skills. I also perform longer sessions based on just one area. For example tackling, competing for the ball and footwork.

How often would you do this type of training in your down time/holidays?
I try to rest from rugby as much as possible, but I always try and get a ball in my hands at least once a week. To keep my eye in, I often play touch in the summer as a way of staying fit and keeping my skills going.

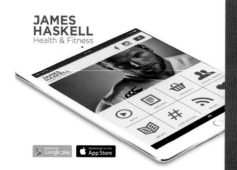

Skills: Competing for the ball

Your partner stands opposite you holding a ball. This drill is done at about fifty to sixty percent intensity as you are not trying to smash each other. It's about the technique more than anything. You can take it up to full contact.

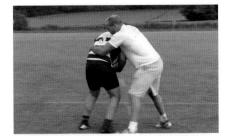

Your partner jogs into you, you force him to ground using an upper body tackle. He obviously only resists a little bit and then goes down to ground. As he hits the ground and goes to place the ball, you show good release (This is very important. If you don't release the tackled player when you are the tackler, you will give away a penalty. Referees are very hot on this) When doing this drill I over-exaggerate this part, making sure I take both my hands off, to clearly show I have released the man. This exaggerated move is known as 'chicken winging'.

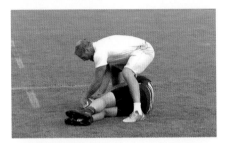

You then get into a low position over the player on the floor and latch onto the ball. You do this while maintaining your own bodyweight and always remaining on both feet. The best way of doing this is to think about three points:

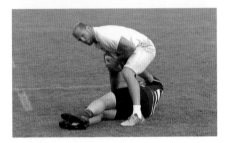

1) Chest right over the ball, so you are not over extended
2) Feet nice and wide giving you a good base
3) Keep as low as possible but with a stable body position

James says:
"You then tug at the ball until you have taken it. It's very important you do this as the referee will want to see you actually steal it."

"You can then reset the drill and go again. Repeat as many times as you want, swapping roles."

"A variation of this is where you hit the floor too as the player goes to ground. Then you bounce back to your feet, show good release and go for the steal. You can advance this drill by performing a low leg tackle, then work back to your feet, show good release and then compete for the ball. You can practice working round and coming through the gate to steal the ball, or if you are the tackler and no ruck has formed (It obviously won't as it's a drill) you are able to get up in whatever position you finish the tackle and take the ball. The ex All Blacks Captain, Ritchie McCaw was a great exponent of this."

STEP 10 RUGBY CORE SKILL DRILLS - PASSING

Skills: Passing

This is an effective but simple drill to work on to develop and improve your passing. This can be done after your main training session of the day, it is not too taxing. However, you can make it tougher.

You need three players to make this work, so try and grab guys as they are walking off the field.

You have two players standing level with each other in a line about ten metres apart. One of them has a ball. The other player is standing close to the guy with the ball.

This is the player who is practicing his passing throughout the drill. He jogs forward and is then passed the ball by the player holding it. The normal rules of rugby apply in this drill. The ball always has to be passed backwards.

As he continues to move forward, he then passes the ball to the other player who is now over ten metres away and standing stationary. He can do this using any style of pass he wants. I suggest you start with a pop pass and as the drill progresses, you then move onto spin passes, out of the back door and rugby league style end-over-end passes.

The player who passed the ball then runs in a loop back round to the guy he has just passed too. He can either do this in a wide arc or something a little more shallow. He can do this fast or slow depending on what you are trying to achieve in the drill. (You can also make this a fitness drill).

As the player runs by the player to whom he passed so now has the ball, he receives the ball back, which he passes onto the first man who passed him the ball. Once a player has completed ten passes off each hand, that is to say the left and right hands, you then swap one of the static passers with the player who has just been working. Every player will have a turn at working. You do this twice through in total.

Once you have all swapped over and done this drill once you can then repeat it a couple more times. Vary the distance of the men you are passing too, but also the quality of pass they feed you with. They can throw it high, low, let it bounce and so forth. However you are still expected to collect the ball and deliver a perfect pass.

Be tough on yourselves. Always ensure you execute a clean and proper pass, making sure you focus on technique.

James says:

"My tips would be always finish with your hands facing towards the man you have passed the ball too. Make sure you look where you pass."

Vary the different types of pass that you use.

Vary the distance you make the pass. I suggest starting at a distance of ten metres but you can shorten or lengthen this subject to accuracy and technique.

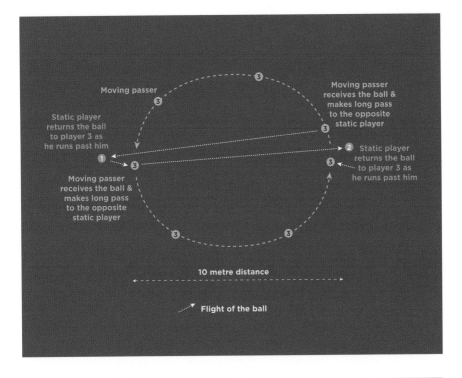

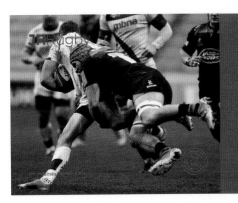

STEP 11 RECOVERY

If you are training hard enough, you are going to get sore. There will also be times when you are injured - it happens to all of us. Recovery can make a huge difference to looking after your body and helping you get the results you need.

Recovery does not just mean sitting on your bottom or lying in bed. You need to get yourself involved in some active recovery. Don't get me wrong sleep and rest will play a huge factor and at times that's the best thing you can do. However, this, as I have suggested, is not the whole story by a long stretch.

Firstly if you have real injury concerns then you need to see a Doctor or at least a Physio. However, If you are just sore then I would look at adopting the following recovery protocols to help you. There is no one miracle method or piece of equipment that will sort you out. Putting a whole range of different things together will make all the difference.

I suggest:

* Ice any strained, bruised or very sore areas
* Look at getting some soft tissue work from a qualified masseur
* Wear compression garments
* Take a Magnesium or Epsom salt bath. Use these after a heavy session but never within forty-eight hours of an upcoming game game.
* Foam rolling - brilliant but don't overdo this.
* MAT-muscle activation treatment. A new approach from specialist trainer Travis Allan. This is something I have introduced in the last two seasons and it has helped me out no end. Have a look at @travisallantt on twitter. It is a type of physical treatment.
* Hot and cold contrast baths, spend one minute in each and finish on a hot bath. You can vary this by using a cold bath and a hot shower for example. Use this kind of recovery after heavy contact sessions. However, avoid doing it after leg weight sessions.
* Eat well – read about our nutrition tips on www.jameshaskell.com
* Always Rehydrate – see prohydrate section on www.jameshaskell.com

Injuries are common when training, but they're mainly due to human error and can be avoided. Common causes of injury include insufficient or no warm-up, lifting with incorrect form, lifting too heavy a weight or not stretching enough throughout the week. Some specific mobility work is essential for a modern rugby player.

Foam rolling is a key tool for anyone preparing to start training or about to undertake training for the first time. Additionally when returning to training after a prolonged absence. You don't want to spend hours doing this or being too aggressive whilst performing the exercise. Six to Eight rolls on each area should be enough.

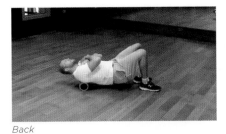

Back

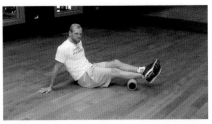

Calves

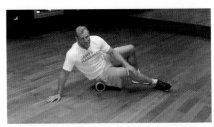

Glutes

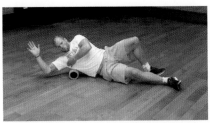

Lats

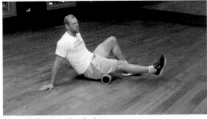

Hamstrings - single leg

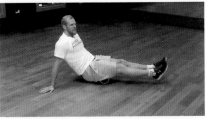

Hamstrings - both legs

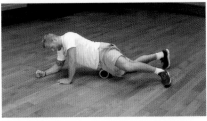

Hips

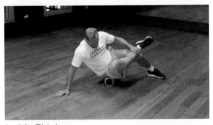

Inside Thigh

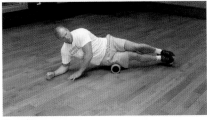

Quads

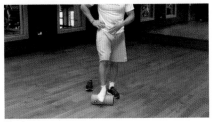

Feet

STEP 12 NUTRITION

Your nutrition is the key to achieving the goals you want. You can do all the training in the world, but if you don't eat properly then you won't adapt as quickly as you should.

James says:
"You need to eat like a rugby player not a cover model."

The best piece of advice I can give when it comes to nutrition is to try to make a couple of small changes and then absolutely stick with them.

An example of a small change is to start eating breakfast, if you don't eat a protein-based breakfast within thirty minutes of waking-up, then look to add this process into your daily diet and meal plan with immediate effect.

Another change would be making sure you eat between three and five good meals every day.
The key principles of your diet should be to be focus on natural, whole foods - avoiding the following like the plague:
• Processed food (junk food, fast food, ready meals etc.)
• Refined foods (white rice, white pasta, white bread, white sugar etc.)
• Fizzy drinks (all are loaded with sugar, so absolutely avoid at all costs)

ON PAGE 80 I have put together a rough plan of the sort of meals and portions you would want to be eating if you have a very heavy training programme. Remember this is not an exact guide for you to follow, as each person's requirements are very different. The following is a suggestion for you to further develop; once you have worked out what works best for you, you need to take the fundamental structure and then tailor it to your own specific needs.

We will create a more focused nutritional guide for you guys to download at a later date. If you look on the website then you will see a number of simple recipes and ideas for you to follow to get the ball rolling.

James says:
"This suggested meal plan is also excellent for size building, but will require a few tweaks to make it suit you as an individual."

If you are a young player looking to put on some size, then you can add in more starchy carbs per meal, as I suggest on the following pages.

Don't try and eat like this right away because you won't be ready for it. You need to gradually make changes.

It's hard work putting on 'good' weight, but absolutely possible if you eat properly with the right amount of carbs, protein, fats and vegetables.

It's important to view diet as one of the most important things you can do for your training, normal health and performance.

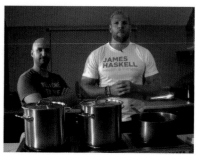

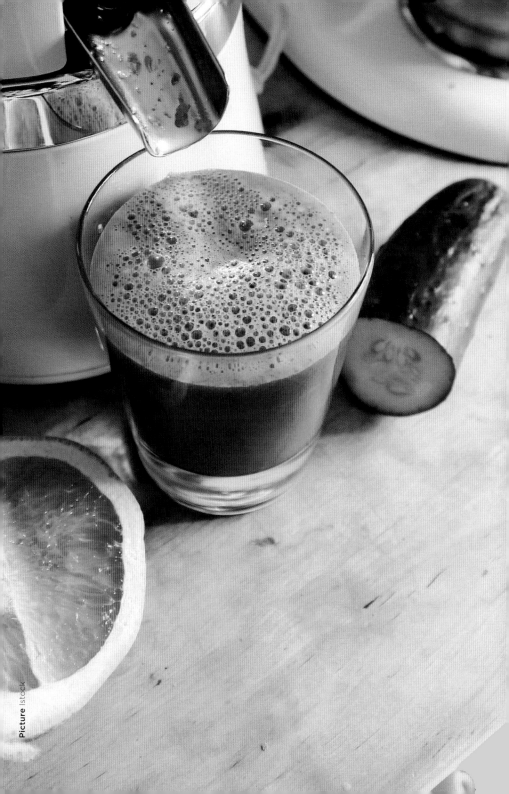

PLATE COMPOSITION

What are Macronutrients?

For those of you who are new to diet and nutrition, the concepts of *macronutrients* (or Marcos for short) and *micronutrients*, are as follows.

Macronutrients are the compounds we eat which provide us with our energy and fuel. These are split into different food groups: protein, fats and carbohydrates. When you read and see talk of your daily macros, it simply means the amount of protein, fat and carbohydrates you will be eating in a day.

Micronutrients are all the vitamins, trace minerals and trace elements which make up the rest of your diet. They have very little if any calorific value but are essential for health, well-being, immune support and function.

James says:
"I would also list water as a key component of your diet. Whilst it does not provide any actual energy, it is essential to all your body processes and without being properly hydrated, you will not be able to perform essential functions."

The 3 Macronutrients:

- **Protein (e.g. meat, poultry, fish, eggs, Greek yogurt)**
  Protein forms the building blocks for your cells. You need it for repair and to build new muscle tissue.
- **Fats (e.g. nuts, eggs, avocado, seeds, coconut oil)**
  Fats are hugely important for the human body, without them the body can't function. They maintain healthy cell membranes, neurone function, absorption of fat-soluble vitamins and the production of hormones.
- **Carbohydrates (e.g. fruit, vegetables, oats, brown rice, potato)**
  Fats and carbs are your body's energy source. Muscle is fuelled by glycogen, aka carbs. So make sure you eat a good, clean amount pre and post training. In order to train well and also achieve size gains, you need to ensure you consume good carbs. Rugby is a sport that requires a lot of fuel, as does trying to build muscle. You need good carbs in your diet.

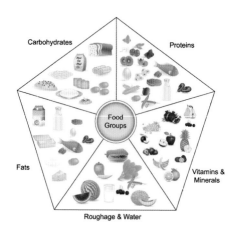

What a rugby player should see when looking down at their plate:

The biggest portion of your plate needs to be made up by a good protein source. For example, chicken, red meat (in moderation), white or oily fish.

Starchy carbohydrates will be your second biggest portion. Things like brown rice, butternut squash, oats, sweet potato etc. *You want to try and stay away from refined carbs. These are things like white pasta, white bread and white rice.*

The third largest portion will be made up of vegetables. You need to aim to get as much variety as you can on your plate throughout the day when it comes to vegetables. *You can eat as much vegetable as you want - don't be afraid of over doing it. Examples would be broccoli, green beans and spinach.*

The smallest segment will be your fats. Your body needs fats and anyone who tells you different is talking nonsense. Fats help metabolise protein as well as reducing adipose (fat tissue in the body). This is key to losing weight and staying in shape. Fats are also a very good energy source which your body needs. They are key for heart health, brain health and joint health.

James says:
"So when you see people reaching for the fat-free products remember they aren't helping themselves, often when fat is removed it is replaced by sugar."

Note – Fat is your friend and sugar most definitely is the number one enemy. Try and avoid sugar at all costs if you can. You don't want to go mad with the fats but examples you should be having are eggs, avocado, nuts, coconut oil and olive oil.

James says:
"One example of fat I like to use a lot of is Coconut oil. I saw it as such an essential tool for my nutritional progression that I brought out my own version called Tagaloa, an organic extra virgin coconut oil. Tagaloa offers multiple fitness, health and dietary benefits - use it as a training supplement, as well as in all forms of cooking and as a substitute for spreads. Anyone really serious about nutrition should have it as a staple in their kitchen."

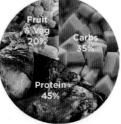

Tagaloa:
- Sugar Free
- Cholesterol Free
- Heat resistant - so much healthier to cook with than olive oil
- Can be taken naturally or added to a pre-training coffee or protein shake
- Coconut oil has a superb combination of fatty acids, which deliver a number of acknowledged health benefits
- It helps develop and supports a positive metabolism but not in isolation from eating the right diet

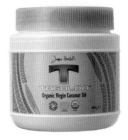

Visit **www.jameshaskell.com** for more information as well as some great recipes

MEAL PLANS

James says:

"Remember – This is loosely based around what I do and is just an example to illustrate what a daily eating plan should look like. My own personal plan is far more extensive than this and fluctuates dramatically depending on whether I am in the off season, pre match, post match etc. What I have given you guys is the most basic plan broken down."

It is not meant to be followed exactly, but rather more as a guide and suggestion, something for you to play around with. Nutrition is trial and error, but you do of course need to follow a simple framework to get the best results.

Taking some time to seek out a good nutritionist will make all the difference. If you have to spend some money it will be well worth it. I am currently working with Aiden Goggins and Glen Matten; these guys are excellent and have helped take my nutrition to the next level. They wrote a great book called the Health Delusion, visit www.aidangoggins.com.

BREAKFAST

If you are eating cereal for breakfast then hang your head in shame. You need to cut this out straight away. There is nothing good in cereal so never buy it. You need to start the day with a protein-based breakfast to help your immune system become engaged and prepared for the day.

Examples of what to eat are (choose 1):

- 2 to 4 Eggs with a handful of vegetables OR one piece of wholemeal bread
- 150g Fish with a handful of vegetables OR one piece of wholemeal bread
- 200g Steak with a handful of vegetables OR one piece of wholemeal bread
- 80g Oats - have this with a handful of nuts and or berries.
  **on training days I would add in the oats as well as all the other proteins

LUNCH

- 200g protein (chicken, fish, lean meat)
- Starchy carbs - 80g uncooked OR 300g cooked (brown rice, butternut squash or sweet potato)
- Unlimited vegetables(you can eat as much of this as you want)
- Small amount fats (add some avocado, eggs or nuts)

AFTERNOON MEAL

- 200g protein (chicken, fish, lean meat)
- Starchy carbs - 80g uncooked OR 300g cooked (brown rice, butternut squash or sweet potato)
- Unlimited vegetables (you can eat as much of this as you want)
- Small amount fats (add some avocado, eggs or nuts)

DINNER

- 200g protein (chicken, fish, lean meat)
- Starchy carbs - 80g uncooked OR 300g cooked (brown rice, butternut squash or sweet potato)
- Unlimited veg (you can eat as much of this as you want)
- Small amount fats (add some avocado, eggs or nuts)

James says:

"It is important to note you can taper down your carb intake towards the end of the day if you have certain body composition goals. This is not necessary for me, so my carbs stay the same."

HYDRATION

Being well hydrated reduces the likelihood of muscular injury, illness, fatigue and will ultimately reduce the chance of regression, or slowed progress, towards your goal.

- Drinking a pint of water upon waking is a great way to re-hydrate.
- Taking a large bottle of water with you to work during the day is good practice- marking lines for how much you should have drunk by a certain time of the day is also a good tip. I have written many times about the importance of hydration. It cannot be underestimated.
- Try to limit intake of standard soft drinks, including diet versions. You can consume high sugar soft drinks intra- or post-workout
- Aim to drink a minimum of between two to five litres of water a day
- Energy drinks should be used when genuinely in need of an energy boost; for example, a pre-workout, during and surrounding training or for a match, or to keep you awake when trying desperately to finish your coursework/ dissertation! Use them very sparingly - they are not great for you.
- As always, factor the calories and sugars from drinks into your daily macros.
- Soft drinks and diet soft drinks are also to be avoided. The medical evidence about their effects are still up in the air. If you can avoid it I would not drink them. If you simply must and have no will-power, then limit your intake to a maximum of one can a day.

James says:
"I would stick to water as your main source of hydration. If that gets boring then you can try water with some fresh lemon juice in it. Lemon juice has been proven to help keep your blood sugar stable. Green tea is good as well. I really like the Tea Pigs Matcha green tea as my hot drink of choice. Tea pigs website www.teapigs.co.uk and their twitter @teapigs."

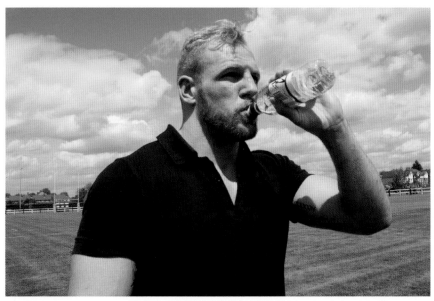

Picture Tickle Media

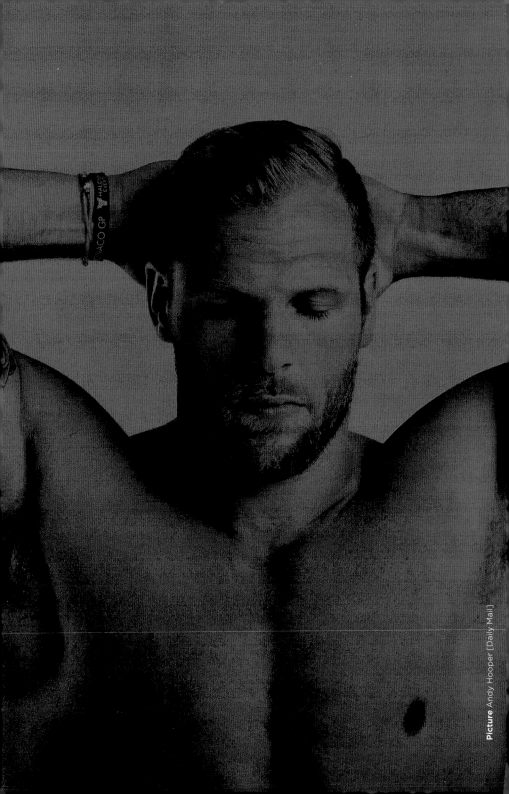

STEP 13 SUPPLEMENTS

James says:
"Ideally, I recommend getting 95% of what you need from balanced, whole, clean foods."

A lot of people, especially young rugby players, reach for supplements first over food. This is completely wrong.

You should spend time and energy on a good diet and please do bear in mind taking protein shakes and creatine is not going to suddenly turn you into a giant.

It's eating large volumes of good healthy protein and carbs which will do that. So stop looking for easy short cuts. I know it is way easier to down a protein shake than cook chicken, brown rice and broccoli. However if you want the gains, then that is what you are going to have to do.

Supplements have their place but it is important you see them as a finishing touch, not the whole process.

The reason behind this is you want to make your digestive system function as well as possible. To do this you should focus on foods that contain the correct enzymes, so they can be digested easily. As a result they are more readily available to the body.

If they don't, they can challenge your immune system, as well as your digestive system. Additionally, the various components of a balanced meal, once digested, work together to perform key functions with essential benefits. In contrast a whey protein shake only contains a simple protein.

If you want to read more about Nutrition then please visit www.jameshaskell. com or visit You Tube - theJamesHaskell

Supplements play an important role in my diet, but ONLY after I have exhausted all possibilities from food. Most of the supplements I take are there to top things up, to help me work on deficient areas (I have had rigorous blood tests to find these out), or help me take on board nutrition quickly, when I don't have food to hand.

I am going to give you some examples of supplements you may want to consider starting to slowly add to your nutrition plan and training protocol but ONLY once you have got on top of your diet.

The supplements will help with performance, recovery and general health, as well as supplementing your diet.

However, never take any supplements, irrespective of source, if the label doesn't clearly display either of these two symbols:

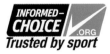 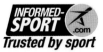

JHEquipment

NEED TO EAT OUT?
ISOBAG MEAL SYSTEM

The Isobag Meal System Range comprises three different styles of USA manufactured, soft-sided, cooler bags, complete with containers and ice packs. Any one of these extremely well-designed bags allows you to plan and enjoy your own healthy nutritious food ,whilst on the go. The Isobag bag is the obvious choice for any Athlete serious about getting their nutrition needs under control and who understand, preparation is essential to get results.

Visit: www.jameshaskell.com/products/equipment/6-meal-iso-bag-full-colour

www.jameshaskell.com

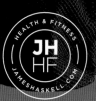

WHEY PROTEIN

Whey is derived from milk; a fast digesting protein source with an excellent amino acid profile that initiates protein synthesis (muscle growth). However if you are lactose intolerant, stick to whey isolates to avoid lactose. Always go for the highest quality brand you can find as a lot of companies add poor quality ingredients or fillers to get more money per tub. I would never buy any products that aren't Informed Sported tested!! Supplements companies who aren't tested don't have to list everything which is in the tub, on the ingredient list. Who knows what you are taking! TAKE ME: Post training sessions when you can't eat a meal within the hour or if you don't have a good food source to hand. Great as a snack when there is no food.

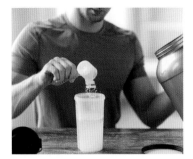

BCAA'S

There are 20 basic amino acids, which are the building blocks of new proteins, however three of these are key to initiating protein synthesis, Leucine, Isoleucine and Valine - otherwise known as Branch Chain Amino Acids. Some argue BCAAS are not completely necessary when on a high calorie diet – but if you have the money, we would recommend taking a BCAA product pre and during your workout to decrease the chance of your body going into a catabolic state (breakdown of muscle tissue for energy) and to promote protein synthesis. TAKE ME: As directed by manufacturer, generally 5-10g pre and during work out

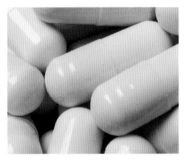

Pictures | Istock

ZMA

Zinc is important for almost all-metabolic processes- especially to protein synthesis and maintenance of a healthy immune system. Magnesium helps regulate electrolyte balance, energy production and neuromuscular function. ZMA is shown to increase growth compounds production and many users (including me) note sensations of deeper sleep when supplementing with it. It's a great aid for recovery. TAKE ME: As directed by manufacturer, generally straight before bed **Remember the key symbols:**

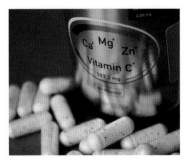

OMEGA 3 FISH OILS

Omega 3 supplements have historically focused on providing a balanced level of these beneficial fatty acids, but increasingly experts in sports nutrition are suggesting obtaining higher levels of EPA could be of greater importance. This is particularly true for high performance sports professionals and active individuals who are looking to aid recovery after intense periods of activity. They are really good for cognitive function (brain health) cardiovascular function (heart health) and joints. TAKE ME: As directed by manufacturer or your nutritionist.

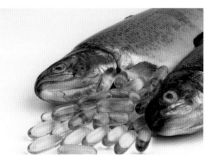

PROBIOTICS

An area which is always neglected when looking at nutritional gains is the health of your gut. If you don't have a healthy digestive system this can affect your immune system, performance and how you absorb nutrients from food. For young players this won't be such an issue, but those older players who haven't eaten well or have put their body under stress could look at trying a high end probiotic to help fix and repair your gut. TAKE ME: As directed by manufacturer or your nutritionist.

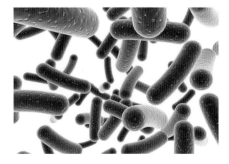

CREATINE

Let's get something straight Creatine is not a steroid and it won't suddenly build you muscle. It is however great for explosive power and is naturally occurring in your muscles already. It will help you work for longer periods and at a high intensity. TAKE ME: As directed by manufacturer or your nutritionist.

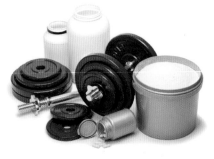

HADES AND HELLA

I didn't use to take pre-trainers before a workout because most of them on the market are untested for athletes and full of rubbish which can cause terrible side effects. I wanted to create something I could take pre-match and pre big training sessions to boost my training, help me focus and work for eighty minutes. So, in conjunction with a top nutritionist, I created my award winning, all natural Informed Sport certified male and female pre-trainer. Hades was in fact voted Best Training Supplement in the 2014 Men's Health Supplement Awards as well as top training product by Functional Sports Nutrition magazine in both 2013, 2014 and 2015.

As you can see from our social media @jameshaskellhf we have had some quite amazing feedback on both products from people using them both .as a pre-trainer, as well as for managing weight loss.

One of the great benefits of Hades and Hella is they don't stop you putting on size, but they will help you put on lean muscle, if you eat the right foods and train well.

To try out any of our James Haskell Health & Fitness supplements please visit: www.jameshaskell.com

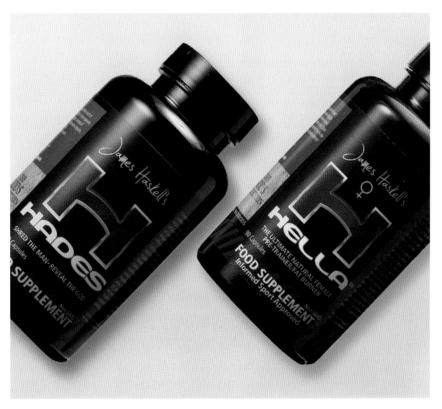

FINAL THOUGHTS

This is the first part of a series of rugby specific packages that we will be publishing.

Within these packages we will be covering off in detail all sorts of areas of the game, including specific fitness and training plans.

So watch out for the next package coming shortly: **Lean Gains Bodybuilding Programme**

If you have any feedback on this package or questions then please tweet us or get in touch.

WHAT'S NEXT?

Stay tuned for our other packages by following our social media links:
Twitter @jameshaskellhf (formerly Jhbodyfire)
Instagram @jameshaskellhf (formerly Jhbodyfire)

If you want to interact with us then please submit your questions using #AskHask and we will either answer the question through one of our video question compilations (available on www.youtube.com/ theJamesHaskell) or tweet you back as soon as we are able.

Enter our Tackle of the Month competition. If you are 12 years and upwards then submit a clip of the biggest tackle you have seen in an amateur school or club game. You can do this either by tweeting us, or emailing it to Jhfitnessblog@gmail.com we will post the clip on our social media channels. Use #tackleofthemonth

You will be entered into a competition to win the chance for tickets to a Wasps game, supplements and a training session with James himself.

Subscribe to our YouTube channel - James Haskell TV or search www.youtube.com/theJamesHaskell - it is full of recipes, fitness tips and humour to keep you going. There are also product reviews, exercise breakdowns and all the inside tips and tricks. We also do James Haskell Live, which is a fully live, Google hangout and YouTube live stream with guest stars from all sports.

Try the Hades and Hella challenge. Twelve weeks to get in the best shape of your life. All you need to do is visit www.jameshaskell.com and purchase a pot of Hades or Hella with the discount code. You then submit a photo of you holding the pot. We give you twice-weekly HIIT sessions for you to perform while taking our supplement. The person who shows the best progress in the twelve weeks will win a training session with James, Beats by Dre kit, supplements and much more. Please visit our instagram to see how amazing some of the results have been. **Get in the shape you deserve now**.

VISIT **JAMESHASKELL.COM** FOR MORE INFORMATION